Drtbalu's OSCE Notes In Otolaryngology

Dr Thiagarajan Balasubramanian

ISBN-13: 978-1467944441

ISBN-10: 1467944440

DEDICATION

I dedicate this book to all My Teachers who have carried me this far on their shoulders

Contents

ACKNOWLEDGMENTS

I wish to place on record my thanks to My Parents who made me exist, My wife and son for making my life worthwhile and My Teachers for shaping my destiny.

1 OSCE AN INTRODUCTION

OSCE (Objective Structured Clinical and Practical Examination) is now the preferred clinical examination modality followed by majority of universities worldwide. This exam pattern is a challenging one for the student as well as examiners. In OSCE a student's clinical / practical skills are put to test. They will be able to fare well only if they had enough clinical exposure during their curriculum period.

Why this change has been brought about? What exactly was wrong with the prevailing examination system?

The conventional Clinical & Practical examination is beset with the following problems:

1. Lack of objectivity

2. Student skill variability

3. Examiner variability

4. The ability to examine a patient and to come to a conclusion is not observed by the examiner

5. The final evaluation score does not give adequate feedback to the candidate

In order to overcome these shortcomings, Harden [1] introduced Objective structured clinical and practical examination (OSCE) in 1979. Gradually OSCE has become more acceptable examination modality due to its objectivity. In his path breaking paper Harden [1] goes on to explain the drawbacks of conventional clinical examination where a student's clinical skill was judged by asking him to examine a couple of cases. According to him it left a lot to chance as the cases were allotted by a draw.

What Exactly is OSCE?

It is an acronym for Objective Structured Clinical and Practical Examination. This system of examination consists of 15 - 20 stations. A student appearing for the exam is expected to spend 4 - 5 minutes inside a station. These stations can be simultaneously run and hence about 15 - 20 students could be examined within 1 hour. The students are expected to complete the task within the station and fill it up in the response sheet provided.

These stations should be carefully planned so that the clinical acumen of the student can be comprehensively tested. All these stations should have observers armed with check lists to assess the student's performance. Some stations are called procedure stations where in the student is expected to perform an examination technique on the patient. These procedure stations should be so designed to test the examination skill of the student.

Advantages of OSCE:

1. The whole examination procedure is objective
2. It integrates teaching and evaluation
3. The sheer variety of cases provides keeps the student's interest intact
4. Interaction level between student and examiner is optimal
5. Patient variability and examiner idiosyncrasies are avoided
6. A large number of students can be evaluated in the shortest possible time

7. It is so flexible that it can be tailored to suit local needs

Limitations of OSCE [2]:

Any system is not fool proof. OSCE examination system also has its own share of limitations. They include:

1. Observer fatigue (Examiner) this is the most serious one
2. It is very difficult to evaluate the overall competency of a candidate in the time allotted. Students are allotted just 4-5 minutes per cubicle.
3. Lot of planning should go in deciding the type of cubicles as they are going to play a vital part in the examination process
4. OSCE is fairly accurate in assessing knowledge and skill levels of undergraduate students. When it comes to post graduate students it fails to assess the student's in-depth knowledge in the subject. [3]
5. More expensive in terms of time and material costs
6. Manual scoring of OSCE is time consuming and tends to become inaccurate

Setting up OSCE Stations

Ideal Clinical examination should have a minimum of 20 cubicles.[1]

Points to be borne in mind while setting up exam cubicles:[4]

1. Questions should be objective in nature
2. Questions should be framed in simple language without ambiguity
3. All the questions framed for a cubicle should be standardized with clear cut weightage for marks.
4. Cubicles should be designed in such a way that it evaluates a student's understanding of the subject, skill of observation, interpretation of signs etc.
5. Examiners should be provided with check list for each cubicle which will enable them to assess the student

Students are expected to spend atleast 5 minutes in each station. Each student is expected to complete the task within the stipulated time and should fill up the response in the sheet provided.

Atleast 20 students can take the test at a time because all these stations can be run simultaneously. Among these stations atleast 2 should be ear marked as procedure stations. These procedure stations will help the examiner to test the examination skill of the candidate.

While setting up OSCE stations two stations should be earmarked as rest stations where candidates can take rest. Refreshments can be provided in that station.

General bed side manners:

Candidates who attend OSCE should be exclusively awarded marks for bed side manners. The following are considered to be really important from patient's point of view:

1. Does the student greet the patient on entering the cubicle?

Greeting a patient is not only a friendly gesture on the part of the examiner, it also instills a sense of confidence on the part of the patient. A patient who is greeted properly tends to cooperate better during clinical examination. It goes without saying that patient's cooperation is an absolute must for any successful clinical examination.

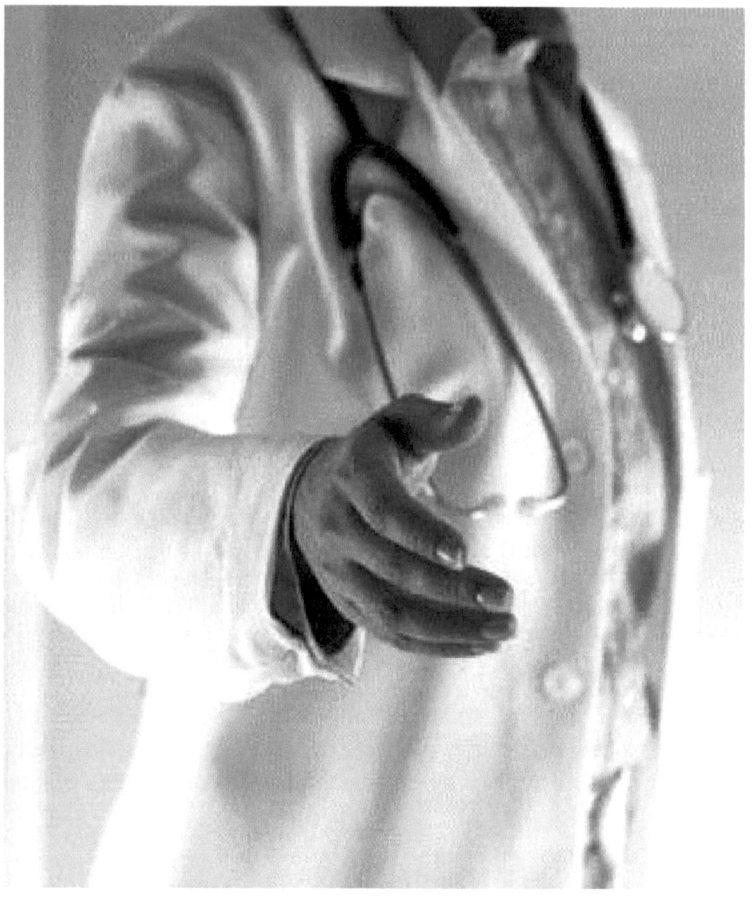

A warm handshake will instill more confidence than a ton of words.

2. The student should wash his / her hands in front of the patient. A basin of water and soap should be provided for this very purpose
3. Does the student explain what he is going to do to the patient in clear terms? Explaining a procedure will ensure better cooperation on the part of the patient. If it is going to be a slightly painful procedure it will ensure that the patient is mentally prepared for the same.

4. Does the student seek permission to examine the patient? This is actually not as a matter of courtesy but it is a must.

5. Does the student provide a screen to maintain privacy? Examiner should look for this aspect of clinical examination. Weightage should be given in terms of marks if a student performs this task.

Timer:

One tutor / skilled assistant is entrusted with the task of maintaining the time. He should be provided with a timer. He will chime a bell as soon as the time allotted to the cubicle is over.

Students should move across the cubicles in only one direction. One examiner should be present at the Procedure station observing the candidate with the check list provided.

Sample check list to evaluate a candidate while performing indirect laryngoscopy:

Station No:

Name of the student:

                                           Yes

No

1. Did the candidate explain the procedure?

2. Was the candidate seated properly?

3. Was the mirror warmed?

4. Which side of the mirror was warmed?

5. Did the patient suffer from pain during The procedure?

6. Did the candidate use sterile gauze to hold The patient's tongue?

Similar checklists should be provided for all cubicles giving observation weightages.

In the scoring checklist the answers can be marked as+ 1 for correct answer, -1 for wrong answer and 0 for not attempting the question.

Two types of OSCE stations can be set.

1. Procedure station – Where the candidate is expected to perform a set of clinical examination
2. Stations containing questions pertaining to the clinical examination performed by the candidate.

Example of procedure station:

Performing Indirect Laryngoscopy on a patient.

In the following stations questions can be asked as follows:

Station 2: Draw a diagram of the findings
Station 3: What could be the probable diagnosis?
Station 4: What could be the stage of the lesion?
Station 5: Which is the confirmatory test?

Tips

For students

OSCE tests the not only the knowledge and clinical skills of the candidate it also tests their attitude and communication skills. All these skills can be perfected by regular practice. There is no substitute for practice and hard work.

Tips regarding appearance

1. *Dress neatly / professionally*
2. *Nails should be clipped one day before examination*
3. *Always stick to your role when you communicate with the patient*
4. *Stay inside the room till the whole allotted time is over*
5. *Don't attempt to make a diagnosis*
6. *Don't skip any procedure*

Communication Tips:

1. Knock the door of the cubicle before you make an entry. This will create a better impression on the patient.
2. Take time to greet the patient warmly with a handshake. Introduce yourself by your name Inform the patient about your status (i.e. student). It is also better to inform the patient about the purpose of your examination
3. Explain in detail the procedure you are going to perform on the patient

4. Always maintain eye contact. This will add sincerity to your purpose
5. Use direct questions to get answers from the patient
6. Be truthful while answering patient's queries
7. Thank the patient when you get your audio signal that time is over

How to tackle History stations?

1. Be calm and composed
2. Always be seated at the eye level of the patient
3. Always begin with broad open questions before moving to the specifics
4. Be patient till the patient answers a question before asking the next
5. Don't cut the patient's answer short. This will leave a bad impression on the patient that you are not keen in listening to his problems.
6. Use nonverbal means to encourage the patient. A smile will go a mile
7. Use follow up questions to elicit correct response from the patient. If the patient says I don't consume alcohol now, follow it up with another question like "When did you have your last drink?" This will probably bring out correct response form the patient.
8. While querying about patient's symptoms focus on eliciting the following 8 attributes:

   Location
   Quality
   Severity
   Duration
   Timing
   Context
   Modifying factors
   Associated signs and symptoms

9. Always mentally summarize before you leave the cubicle

How to tackle Clinical examination stations?

1. Always ensure that you carry examination instruments / whether all instruments necessary for the examination are present inside the cubicle.
2. Always wash your hands in the basin provided before beginning the clinical examination
3. Always discuss the procedure with the patient before starting the examination
4. Patient should be informed about the exact purpose of the examination
5. Always help the patient on and off the examination table

Otology Clinics

1. Look at the patient's face. Examine his right external auditory canal. Name the probable disorder.

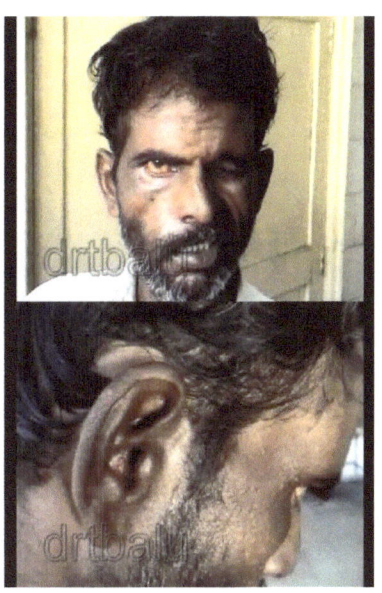

Loss of wrinkling of right forehead +

Inability to close right eye +

Deviation of angle of mouth to the left +

Lower motor neuron type of facial palsy on the right side.

Blisters seen in the external right external auditory canal

Name the syndrome: Ramsay Hunt syndrome

Name the causative organism : Varicella zoster virus

Name the areas where rashes can be seen in this syndrome: Anterior 2/3 tongue, soft palate, external auditory canal and pinna

Name the various eye care procedures that should be followed in a patient with Ramsay Hunt syndrome.

Wearing of eye glasses and use of moisturizing eye drops. The intention is to prevent exposure keratitis

2.

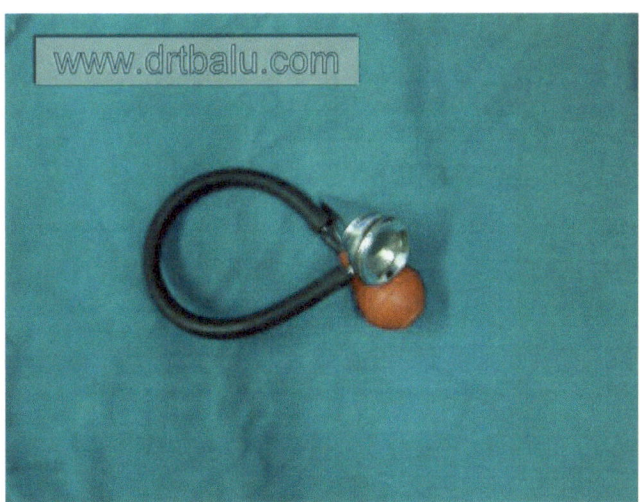

Name the instrument shown in the picture

Mention its uses

It is a siegle's pneumatic aural speculum.
It is used to examine the ear drum, test its
mobility. It gives a magnified vision.
Magnification factor is about 2.5 times.

3. Given below is the picture showing otoscopic findings of a patient's ear. Describe the findings.

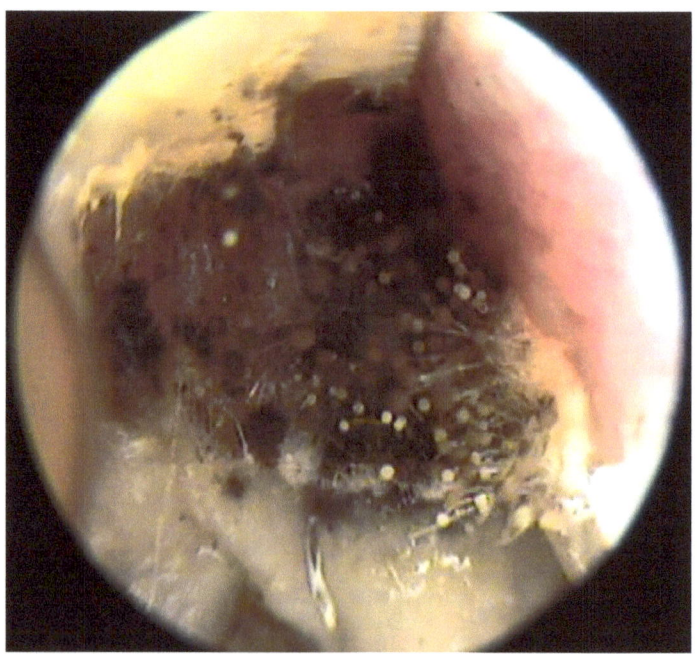

Cotton wool like mass seen in the external auditory canal. This cotton wool structure could be seen interspaced with black spots. The diagnosis is otomycosis. Whitish cotton wool patches are caused by candida and black spots are caused by Aspergillus niger.

8. What could be the complaints with which patient will present?

Itching sensation in the ear
Pain in the ear due to otitis externa
Serous discharge from external auditory canal

Blocking sensation

9.

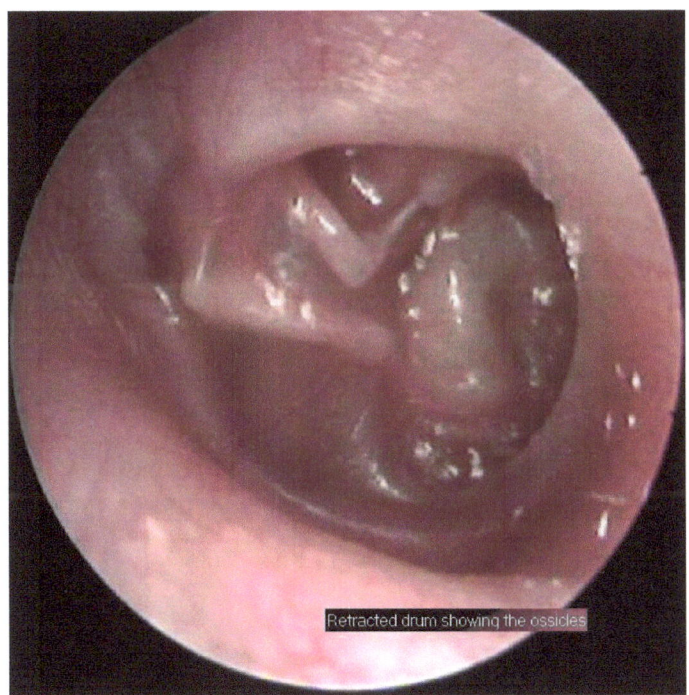

Describe the otoscopic findings seen in this patient.

Loss of light reflex
Prominence of handle of malleus
Loss of ear drum mobility on siegelization
Retracted ear drum

These are all classic features of adhesive otitis media

Additional resources online
(http://www.drtbalu.co.in/retrac_pock.html)

10. Name the numbered structures in the figure

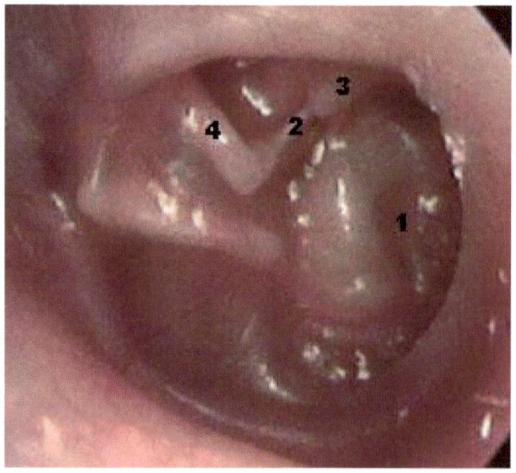

1 – Round window

2 – Stapedial tendon

3 - Pyramid

4 – Long process of incus

11. Name the causes of bilateral retraction of ear drum

   Nasopharyngeal carcinoma

   Following adenotonsillectomy due to damage to Eustachean tube

   Cleft palate

   12. Comment on the ear discharge of this patient. Frame your comments as per otoscopy findings

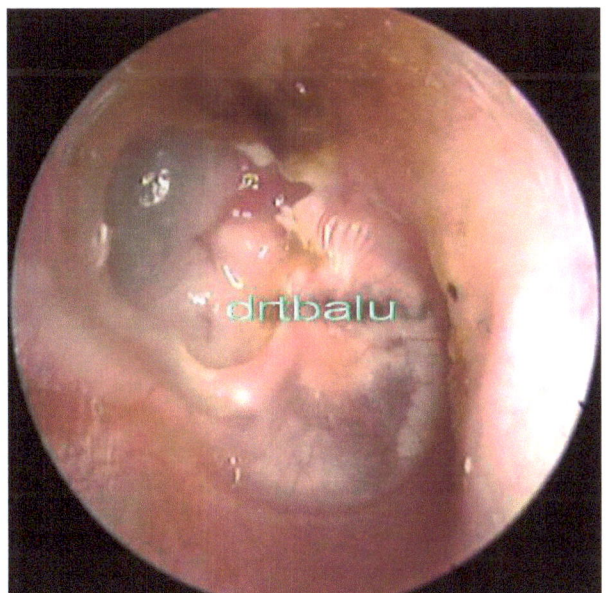

   Scanty

   Foul smelling

   Sometimes blood tinged

Attic cholesteatoma

Online resources for further reading
(http://sites.google.com/site/drtbalusotolary ngology/otology/cholesteatoma)

13.
Name the condition seen in the ear drum. Enumerate three causes for it.

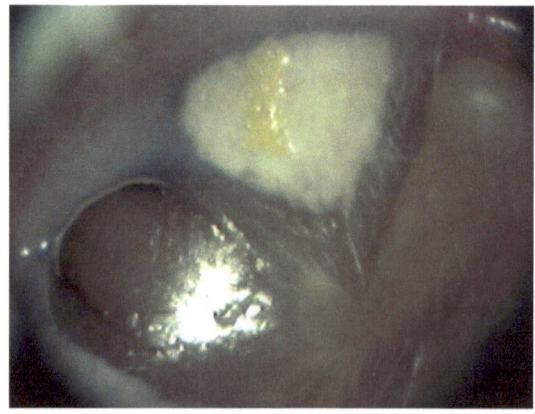

It is tympanosclerosis.

Causes for tympanosclerosis include:

Resolved otitis media

Trauma

Iatrogenic (Grommet insertion)

Online resources for further reading (http://www.drtbalu.com/tympanosclerosis.html)

14. 65 years old man

Known diabetic for 15 years on poor glycemic control

c/o pain left ear - 1 month

Blood stained discharge from left ear - 1 month

Tragal tenderness left side - 15 days

Inability to close left eye - 10 days

Otoscopic finding:

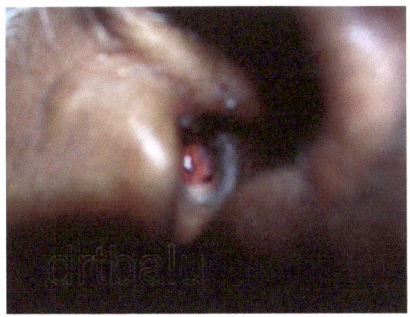

a.   What could be the probable diagnosis?

b.   Name the causative organism

c.   Name the drug of choice for treatment

Malignant otitis externa

Pseudomonas aeruginosa

Carbenicillin / IV generation cephalosporins

15. Enumerate the Levenson's criteria for diagnosis of Malignant otitis externa.

Refractory otitis externa

Severe nocturnal otalgia

Purulent otorrhoea

Granulation tissue in external canal

Growth of pseudomonas organism from cultures of external canal

Presence of diabetes mellitus / immunocompromised state

Further read:
(http://www.drtbalu.com/Malignantotitisexterna.html)

16. 5 years old child

C/O excruciating pain right ear – 6 hours

H/O URI – 2 days

Otoscopy findings:

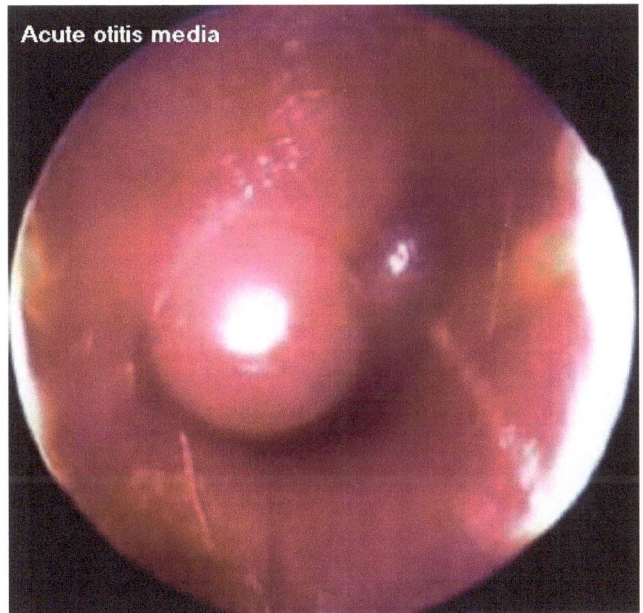

What is the diagnosis?

Name the various stages of this disorder.

Acute otitis media

Stages of acute otitis media: Stage of hyperemia, Stage of exudation, Stage of suppuration and Stage of resolution.

17. Name the surgery performed in AOM. Enumerate its indication

Myringotomy

Surgery is indicated in patients who don't respond to medical management for 48 hours.

18. Post-surgical otoscopic findings of a patient with AOM

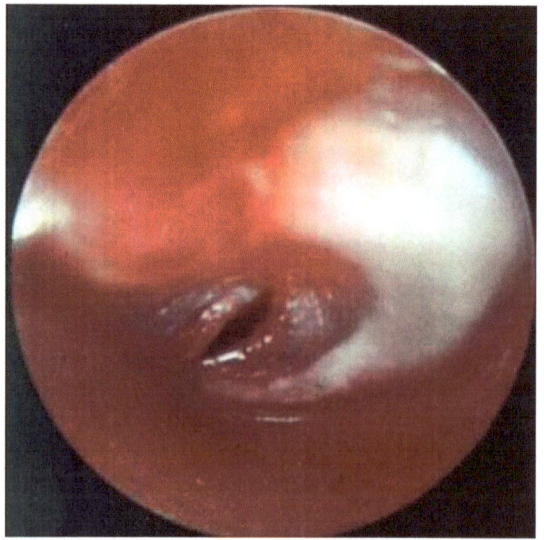

Name the instrument used in this surgical procedure
Name the possible complications of this surgery

Myringotomy knife

Complications include:

a. Dislocation of incus
b. Injury to chora tympani nerve

c.   Persistent perforation

Further read. Online resources
(http://www.drtbalu.co.in/asom.html)

19.   50 years old female patient came with c/o

Pulsatile tinnitus – 3 years in right ear
Hard of hearing right ear – 2 years

Otoscopic findings:

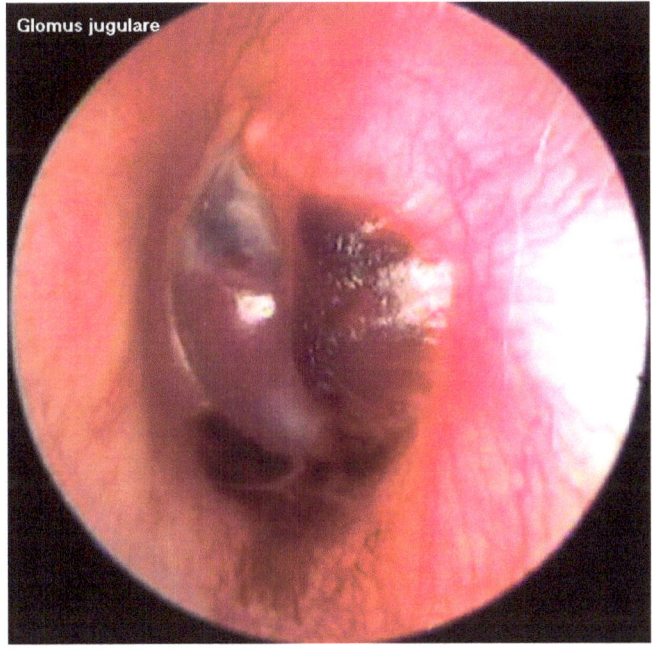

Pulsatile reddish mass seen behind intact ear drum
Name the probable lesion
Name the classic sign seen in the otoscopic image
What is the role of siegelization in this patient?

Glomus Jugulare

Rising sun shine (the red mass seen behind the ear drum)

On siegelization the reddish mass behind the drum blanches (Brown's sign)

20. Name the clinical features of Glomus jugulare:

Deafness

Tinnitus

Imbalance

Otorrhoea

Facial palsy

Endocrine symptoms

Headache

Visual disturbances

21.

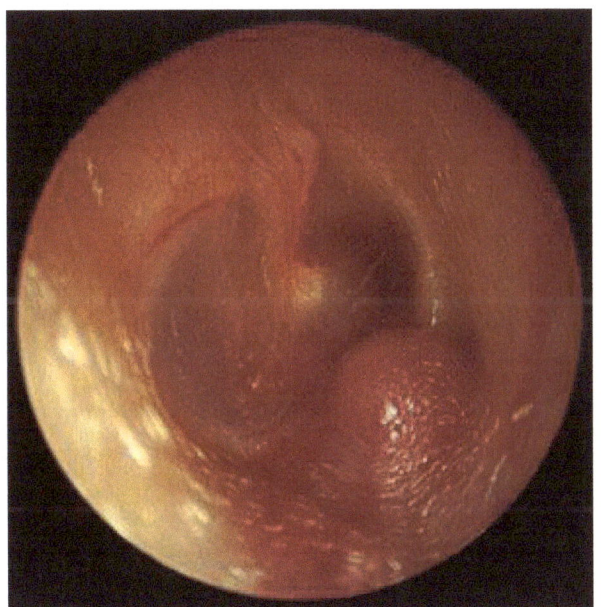

This is a red drum. Probable causes of this problem include:

Aom – Associated with otalgia

High jugular bulb (Normal variant. CT scan shows normal jugular bulb area)

Glomus jugulare associated with the classic signs discussed above

Further read online:
(http://www.drtbalu.co.in/glo_jug.html)

22.

40 years old male patient

C/O swelling behind left ear – 7 days

Pain over left ear – 4 days

H/O discharge from the same ear – 8 years

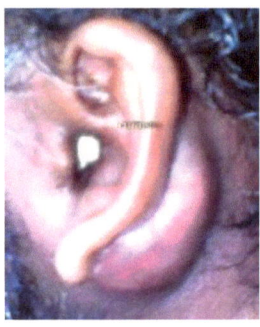

What could be the differential diagnosis?

1.   Subperiosteal abscess
2.   Suppurative retroauricular lymph node

23.

30 years old male patient came with C/O

Pain right ear – 1 week

Blocking sensation right ear – 10 days

Mild discharge from right ear – 1 week

Otoscopy findings:

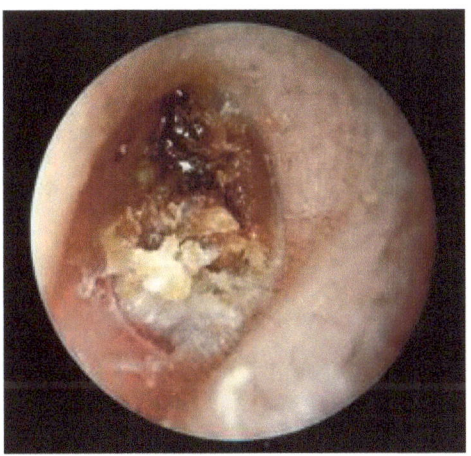

Enumerate otoscopic findings
Mention the probable diagnosis
Mention in brief pathophysiology of this disorder

Whitish mass mixed with wax could be seen in the external auditory canal
External canal appears to be widened
Probable diagnosis – Keratosis obturans
Keratosis obturans occur due to faulty migration of external canal skin.
This movement occurs in a reverse direction in these patients i.e. towards
The ear drum instead of away from it.

Further read
(http://sites.google.com/site/drtbalusotolaryng ology/otology/keratosis-obturans)

24.

Perform three finger test on this patient.

Greet the patient first

Explain the procedure

Reassure the patient

Three fingers are used to perform this test.

Middle finger is used to apply pressure over the well of the concha - Tenderness in this area indicates tenderness over the antral area

Index finger is used to apply pressure over mastoid process - Tenderness indicates mastoiditis

Thumb is used to apply pressure over mastoid tip - Tenderness indicates mastoid emissary vein thrombophlebitis

25.

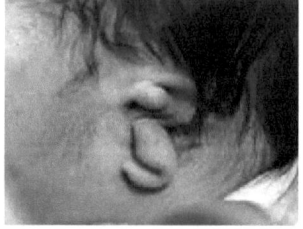

Name the type of pinna seen here

Name some drugs which when ingested during pregnancy would cause this condition

Microtia

Warfarin, Folic acid antagonists like methotrexate and aminopterin

Additional read
(http://www.drtbalu.com/microtia.html)

26.

22 year male patient came with c/o swelling over right pinna - 4 days

Mild pain ++

No h/o fever

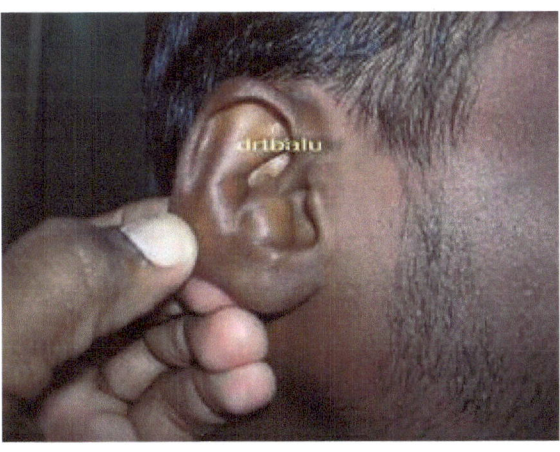

Name the possible pathology

How will you manage this condition ?

Aural seroma

Needle aspiration with application of compression dressing to   prevent reaccumulation.

27.

Perform Unterberger test on this patient

Narrate the aim of this test

What will happen if the patient has a paralytic labyrinthine lesion ?

What will happen in the presence of an active irritative lesion ?

1. Greet the patient.

2. Explain the procedure to the patient / take his consent

3. This test aims to reduce proprioceptive input

4. The patient will rotate to the side of a paralytic labyrinthine lesion

5. In the presence of an active and irritative lesion the patient cannot perform this test.

Procedure:

The patient is asked to stand with eyes closed and hands outstretched.

He is instructed to march on the spot.

28.

30 year old male came with swelling & tenderness over right parotid area - 3 days duration

H/O Right ear discharge on and off - 3 months.

How could the infection from ear spread to the parotid gland ?

Spread of infections from mastoid and vice versa can occur through fissures of santorini.

This fissure is present over the cartilaginous portion of the external auditory canal.

29.

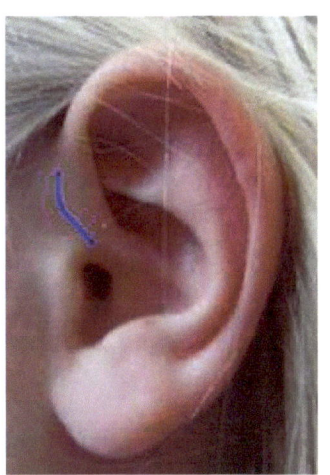

Name the incision

Why is this area preferred ?

This is endaural incision used for mastoidectomy.

This area is devoid of cartilage.

30.

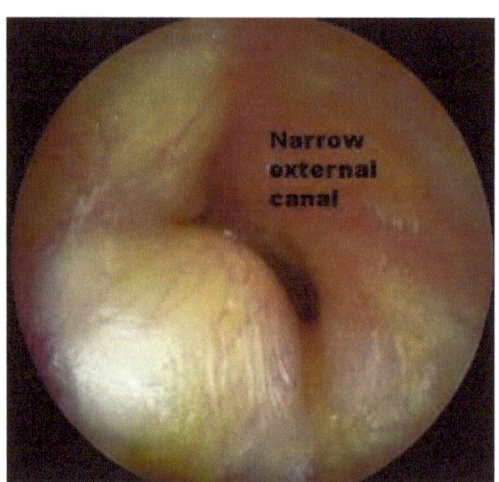

Why is this external auditory canal narrow ?

What could be the cause ?

What could be the clinical problems faced by the patient ?

What surgery should be performed in this patient ?

Exostosis of external auditory canal.

It is common in swimmers.

These patients have conductive deafness, cerumen impaction.

Cerumen impaction is caused by abnormal self cleansing mechanism of the skin lining external canal in these patients.

Canalplasty

31.

24 years old male patient

C/O Ringing sound in his left ear - 2 years
Hard of hearing left ear -8 months

Otoscopy finding:

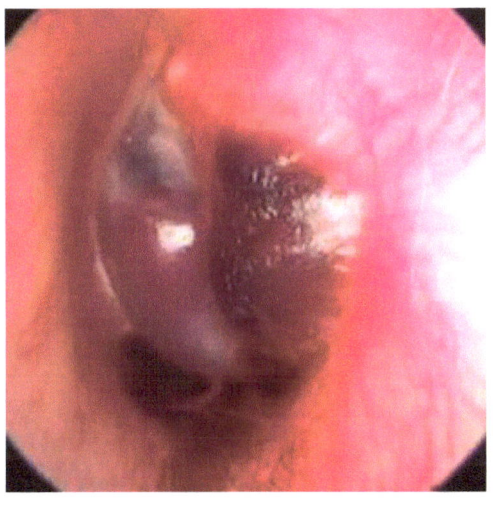

What could be the possible diagnosis ?

Which cell gives rise to this condition ?

Glomus jugulare tumor

Paraganglia cells

32.

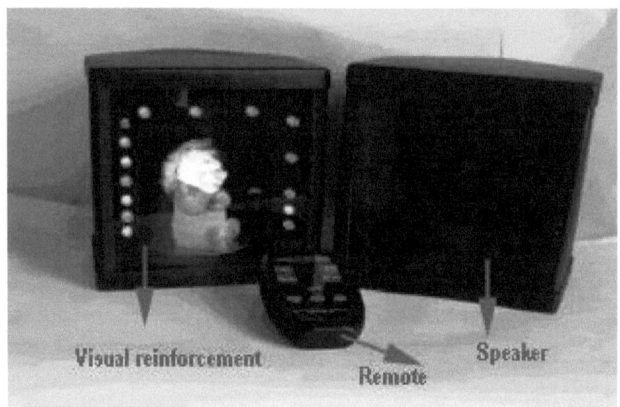

Name the instrument ?

What is its use ?

It is a visual response audiometer.

It is used to screen infants for hearing disabilities.

33.

30 years old female patient came with c/o:

1. Recurrent fractures of Metatarsal bones

2. HOH both ears - 8 years

3. No h/o ear discharge

4. Puretone audiogram showed 60dB conductive deafness both ears

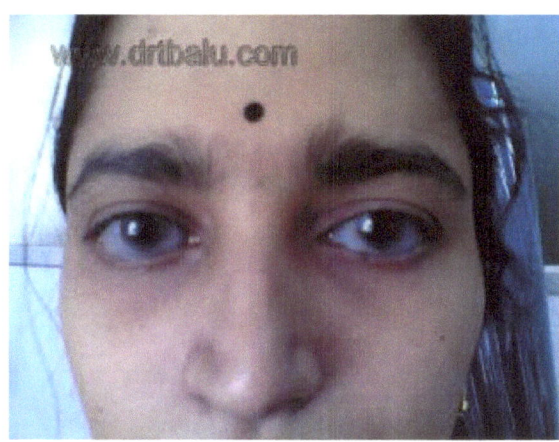

Image shows the patient.

What could be the possible diagnosis?

The patient shows blue sclera both eyes.

Possible diagnosis is osteogenesis imperfecta.
It is characterized by brittle bones, blue sclera and fixation of foot plate of stapes.

34.

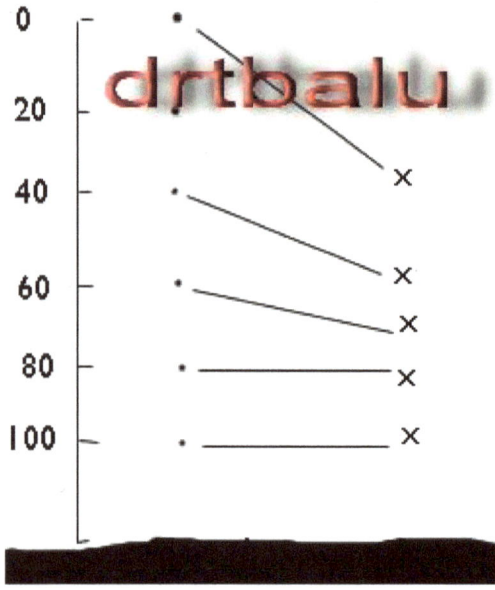

What is this ?
Comment on this diagram

It is a laddergram of ABLB test (Alternate loudness
balance test)

This laddergram indicates complete recruitment..
Recruitment is common in cochlear deafness. It is not
seen in retrocochlear deafness.

35.

30 years old male patient came with complaints of foul smelling discharge from his right ear - 10 days.
He also complained of mild pain in the right ear. Itching ++ in right ear.

Otoscopy picture is seen below:

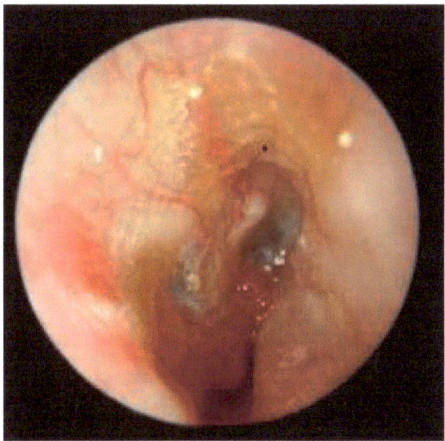

Comment on the otoscopy picture. What could be the possible diagnosis?

Otoscopy picture shows a tongue of granualtion tissue over the inferior quadrant of the ear drum.
Ear drum is probably intact.
Diagnosis - ? Myringitis granulosa.

MOBILITY OF EAR DRUM SHOULD BE TESTED TO RULE OUT EAR DRUM PERFORATION.

36.

12 years old female patient came with c/o swelling in front of right ear 4 years duration.

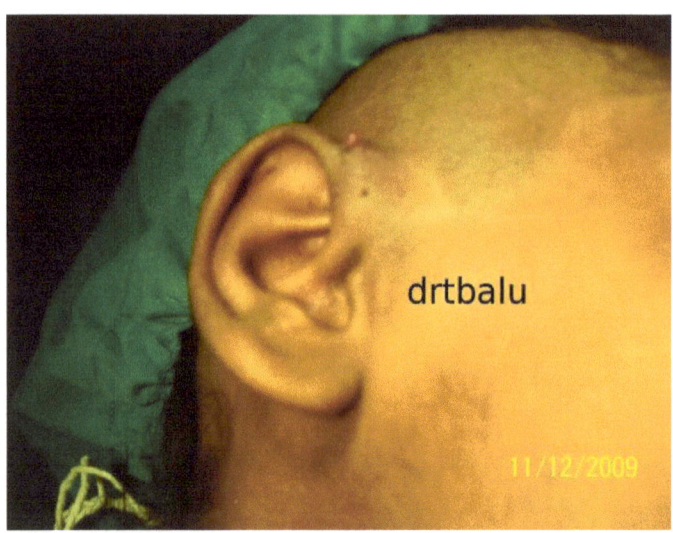

What could be the probable diagnosis?

What complications could it cause?

What is the ideal treatment modality?

Name some syndromes associated with it?

The diagnosis is infected preauricular sinus.

It can get infected and abscess formation in that area can occur.

Surgical removal of the sinus tract completely is ideal.

Branchio oto renal syndrome, Branchio oto urethral syndrome, Branchio otic syndrome, cat eye syndrome, Trisomy 22

Should all patients with preauricular sinus undergo ultrasound abdomen?

No not necessary. To identify those patients who require abdominal ultrasound Wang's criteria should be used. Wang's criteria include:

1. Presence of another malformation / Dysmorphic feature

2. Family history of deafness

3. Malformations involving pinna

4. Maternal history of gestational diabetes

37.

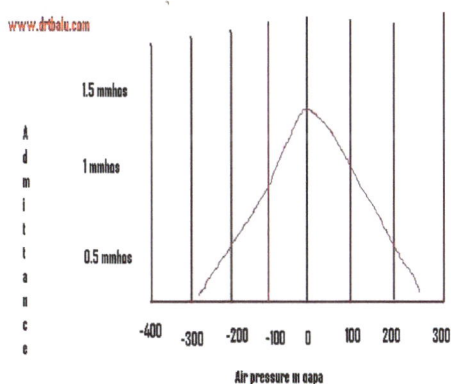

What is this image?

It is a tympanometry recording showing Type a curve.

What does this curve indicate?

This curve Suggests normal middle ear function. The compliance peak occur between -150 - +100 dapa. The value of compliance ranging between 0.2 - 2.5 millimhos. This type of curve is also known to occur in early stages of otosclerosis.

38.

Name the cranial nerves whose functions can be tested by using Impedance audiometry:

7th cranial nerve and 8th cranial nerve functions can be tested by performing this investigation.

39.

30 years old female patient came to the OPD with c/o:

Hard of hearing both sides – 4 years
Tinnitus on and off left ear – 6 months

O/e:

Ear drum on both sides appeared normal. They also showed normal mobility on siegalization.

Given below is the audiogram of the patient:

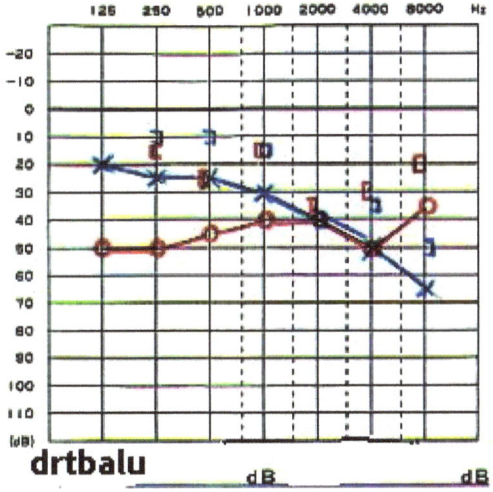

What could be the probable diagnosis?
What do you see in the audiogram?

This patient is probably suffering from otosclerosis.

The audiogram shows carharts notch. It is classically seen in bone conduction audiogram of patients as a dip centered around 2000Hz.

40.

12 years old boy came with complaints of:

Swelling behind left ear - 5 days
Pain left ear - 7 days
H/O URI ++

O/E:

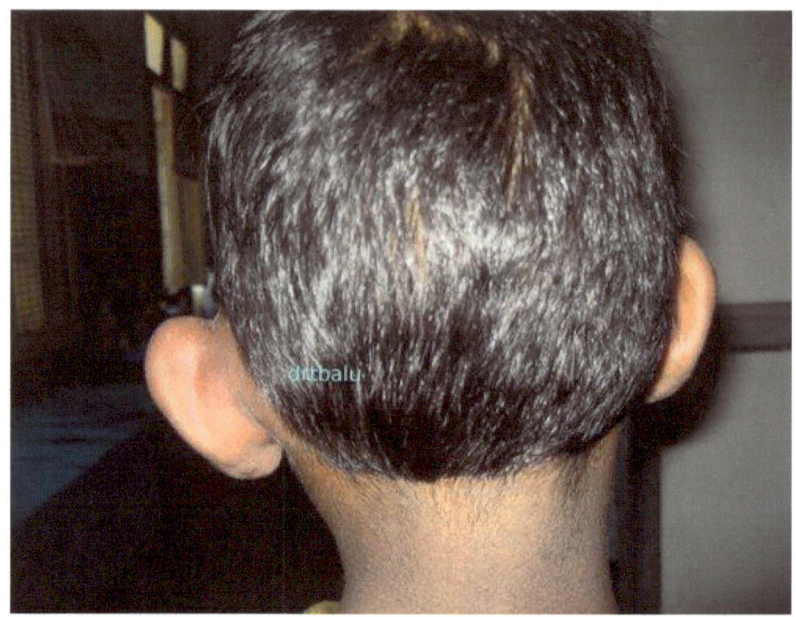

What could be the probable differential diagnosis?
Can you name the most probable diagnosis? How?

DD:

1. Subperiosteal abscess
2. Otitis externa

Out of these two subperiosteal abscess is more probable because:

1. The post aural groove is not obliterated on the right side, which would be if the patient has acute otitis externa.
2. Patient gives history of URI.

2.

Otoradiology

1.

View this x-ray

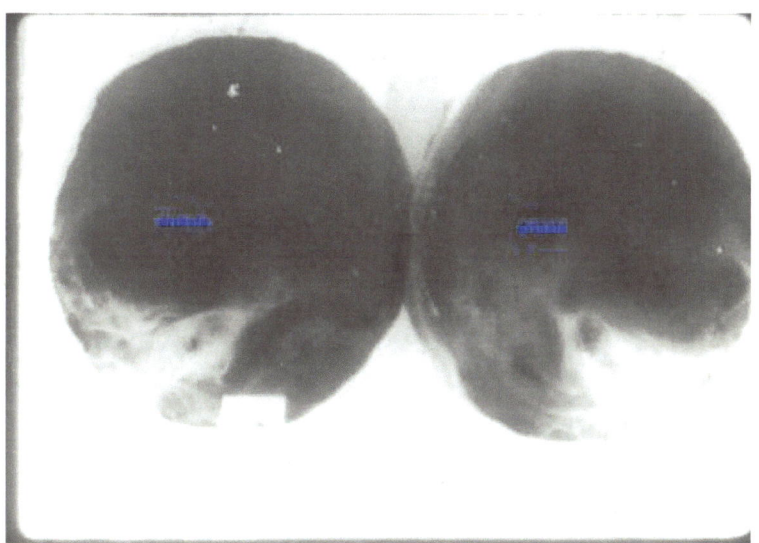

1. Name the view

2. Write down the differential diagnosis

X-ray both mastoids Laws view (lateral oblique)

Differential diagnosis:

1. Large antral cell - This is usually bilateral

2. Cholesteatomatous cavity - Radiologically this cavity will be surrounded by a rim of sclerosis

3. Operated cavity - Pt will give h/o mastoid surgery. The cavity margins will be irregular and will not show sclerosis

4. Secondaries

5. Multiple myeloma

6. Tuberculosis

7. Eosinophilic granuloma

2.

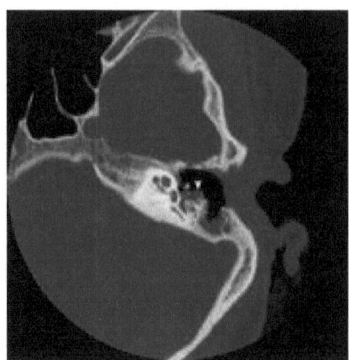

Read this CT scan

This is a CT scan of temporal bone.

Soft tissue shadow seen occupying the middle ear cavity, it even extends to involve mastoid air cell system.

Possible diagnosis – Cholesteatoma

\

3.

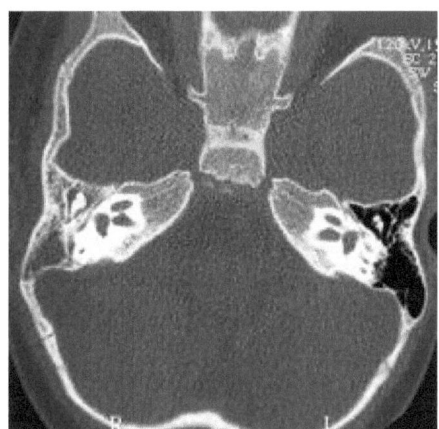

1. What view is this CT scan ?

2. What could be the probable diagnosis ?

This is a plain CT axial view of temporal bone.

It shows sclerosis of mastoid air cells on the right side - possibly due to mastoiditis

Mastoid air cell pneumatization is normal on the left side

4.

Read this CT scan temporal bone axial view

What could be the clinical manifestation seen in this patient ?

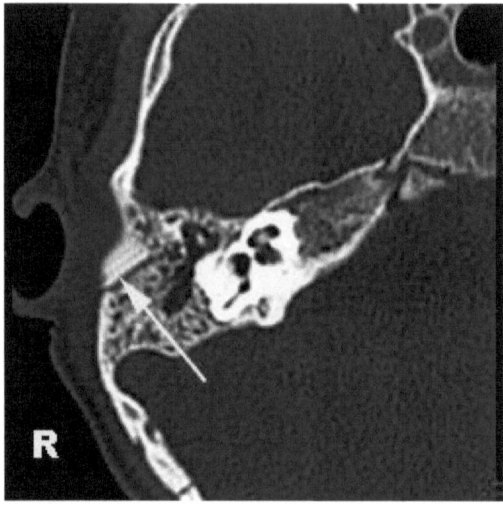

This CT scan temporal bone axial view shows longitudinal fracture of temporal bone

Haematoma could be seen filling the middle ear cavity

These patients commonly manifest with conductive deafness due to the presence of hematoma in the middle ear, or disruption of ossicular continuity.

5.

Comment on the CT displayed

Describe the cochlear deformity

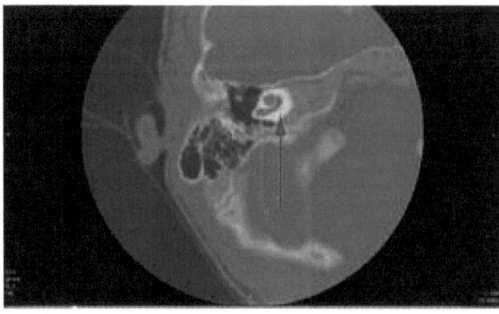

This is a HRCT of temporal bone, axial view.

It shows a deformed cochlea with less than 2 1/2 turns. This is a classical feature of Mondini deformity

6.

Shown below is the CT scan of a patient before cochlear implant procedure.

Identify the pathology

Discuss its relevance to cochlear implant procedure

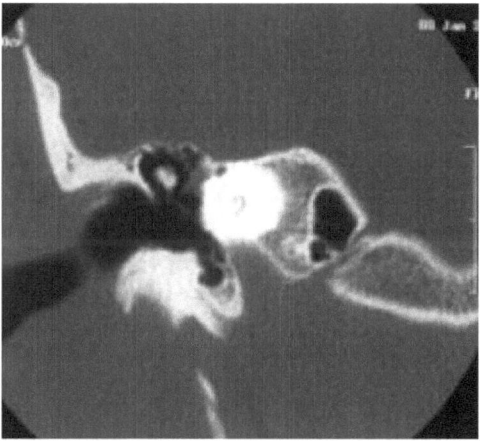

This is a HRCT of temporal bone showing ossified labyrinth. (Labyrinthitis ossificans).

In these patients since the round window is totally obliterated due to ossification it will be difficult to place the cochlear implant electrode.

A third window will have to be drilled for placement of cochlear implant electrodes.

7.

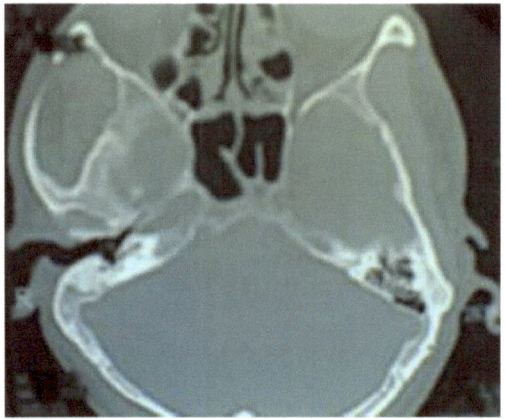

Name the pathology seen in this CT scan.

What type of hearing loss this patient will have ?

This is a axial CT of temporal bone.

It shows atresia of left external auditory canal

Cochlea appears normal

Deafness could be conductive in nature

8.

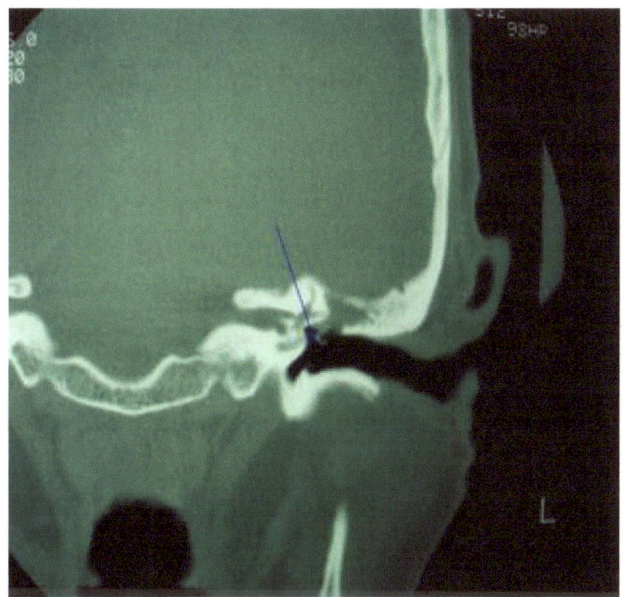

This 30 year old patient had C/O left ear discharge - 5 years

Discharge was scanty, blood tinged and foul smelling

Axial CT (plain) of temporal bone is displayed

1. Identify the pathology

2. Why is the discharge foul smelling ?

This CT shows erosion of the outer attic wall on the left side.

This could most probably be due to cholesteatoma.

Foul smelling discharge is caused due to bone erosion

9.

10 year old boy with h/o grommet insertion left ear one month back.

C/O pain in the left ear

Patient underwent CT scan

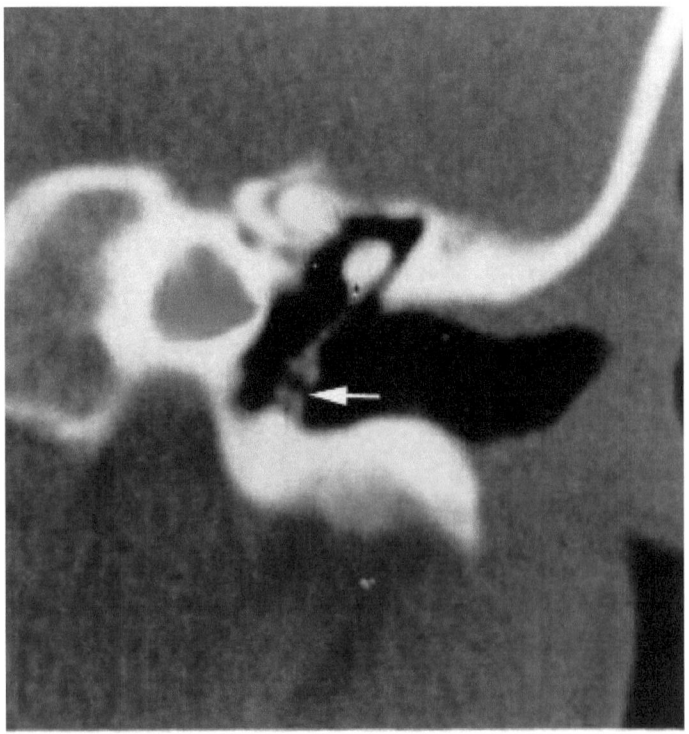

Identify the structure shown by the arrow

Ear drum can be clearly seen.

There is a communication between the external canal and middle ear cavity as pointed by the white arrow.

The site of this communication indicates that it could be the site of grommet insertion

10.

20 year old male patient had c/o Hard of hearing in right ear

There were no other otologic complaints like tinnitus / vertigo / facial nerve dysfunction etc

There was a bony mass arising from the medial aspect of external auditory canal on the right side

The ear was completely dry

CT scan temporal bone :

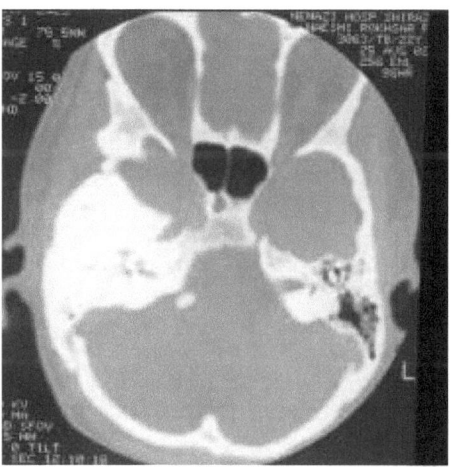

Name the view

Describe the saliant features of this CT scan

What could be the probable diagnosis

This is Axial CT scan plain of both temporal bones

There is a well demarcated bone dense tumor involving the right temporal bone

Middle ear cavity obliterated

No bony erosion of petrous apex

Probable diagnosis - Benign osteoma of right temporal bone

11.

15 years old boy presented with c/o:

1. foul smelling ear discharge left side - 15 days

2. Fever - 2 days

3. Intense headache - 2days

4. There was tenderness / oedema over left mastoid process

Temperature chart:

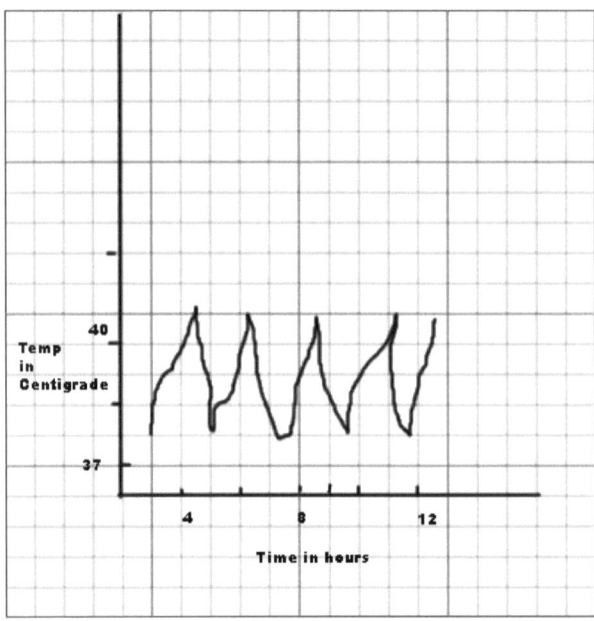

MRI scan:

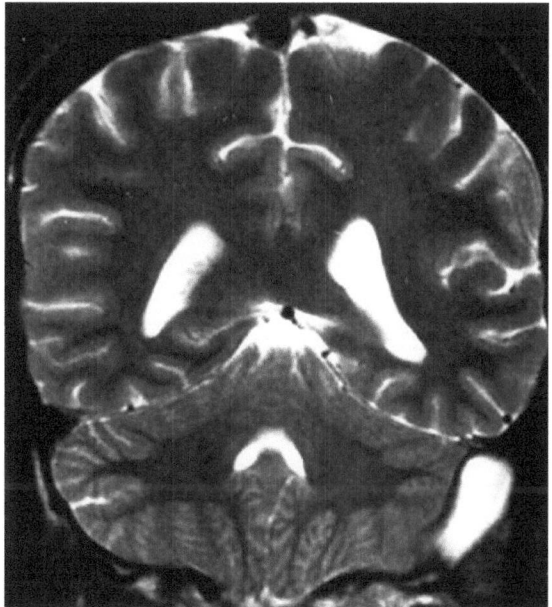

Name the type of temperature chart

Comment on MRI scan of the patient

What could be the probable diagnosis ?

Temperature chart shows classic picket fence appearance. The temperature does not touch normal at any given point of time.

MRI shows clot in the left lateral sinus.

Diagnosis - Otogenic lateral sinus thrombosis

12.

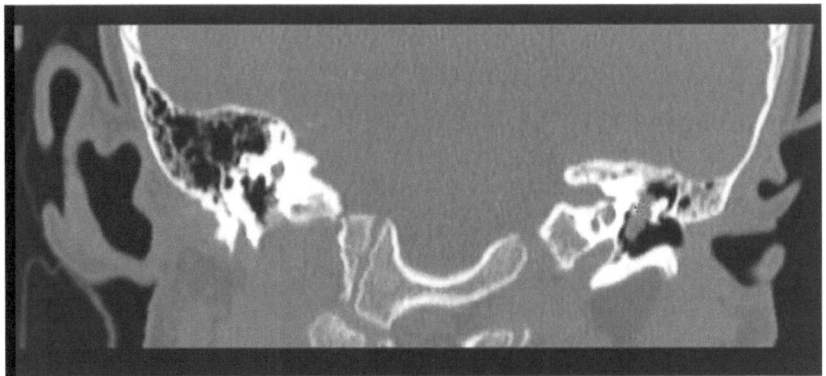

30 year old female patient came to the OPD with C/O mild hard of hearing right ear - 3 years

She gave no h/o ear discharge / pain

O/E: Ear drum was found intact in the right ear.
Mobility was also normal.

CT scan of temporal bone was taken

Comment on the CT scan

This is a CT scan of temporal bone.
Soft tissue shadow is seen occupying the middle ear cavity close to the long process of incus.
Possible diagnosis is cholesteatoma ?? congenital.

Derlacki and Clemis criteria for the diagnosis of congenital cholesteatoma:

1. The patient should not have previous episodes of middle ear disease

2. Ear drum must be intact and normal

3. It is purely an incidental finding

13.

Comment on the CT brain displayed.

Which condition commonly cause this problem?

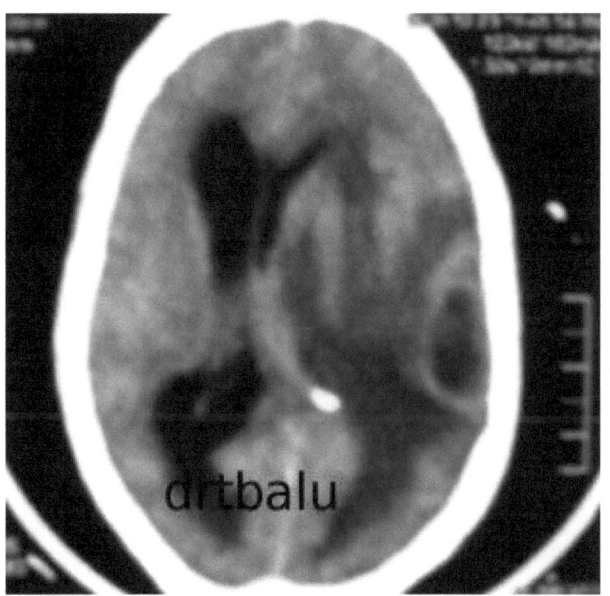

This CT scan brain shows hypodense mass in the right temporal lobe. This mass is surrounded by thickened capsule. Probable diagnosis is temporal lobe abscess. Commonest cause of temporal lobe abscess is chronic suppurative otitis media.

14.

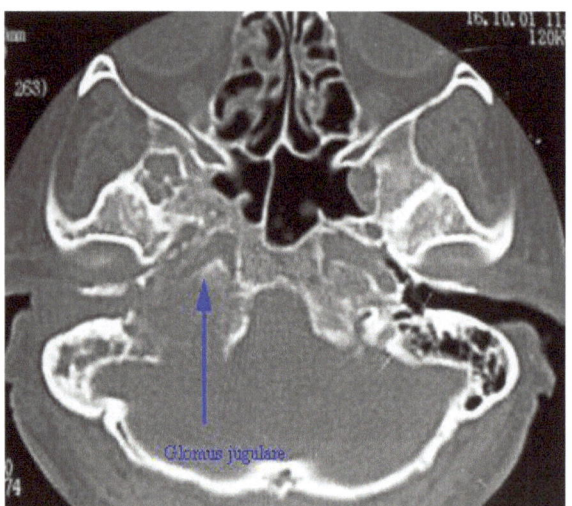

Shown here is the CT scan (axial cut) of petrous bone area showing glomus jugulare as marked there. How do you differentiate it from high jugular bulb and aberrant internal carotid artery?

In patients with glomus jugulare and high jugular bulb the jugular fossa is enlarged. But in glomus jugulare the cortex of the jugular fossa appears eroded while in patients with high jugular bulb this erosion is not seen.

To rule out aberrant carotid artery a coronal CT of temporal bone is a must. If the carotid canal is normally placed then glomus tympanicum should be considered, whereas if the same is placed laterally then aberrant internal carotid artery is a good diagnostic possibility.

15.

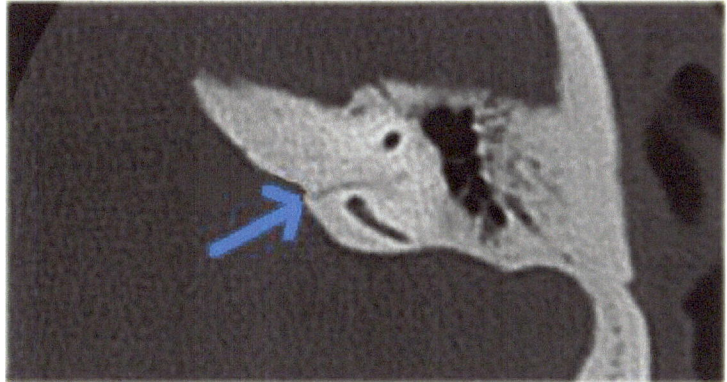

Name the structure pointed out by the arrow.

This is petromastoid canal also known as subarcuate canal. It connects the mastoid antrum with cranial cavity. It houses subarcuate artery and vein. It may be 0.5 mm wide and may be confused with that of fracture line.

16.

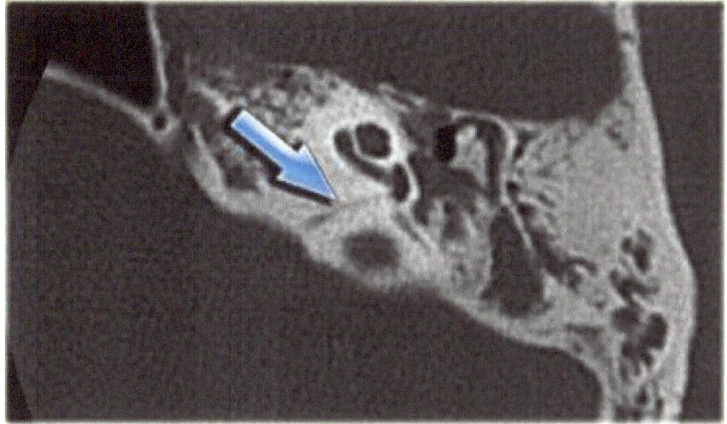

Name the structure pointed out by the arrow.

It is a cochlear aqueduct. It connects perilymph with the subarachnoid space.
This canal runs towards the cochlea in the same direction

as that of internal acoustic meatus, but
more caudally. It is through this duct infections from brain
reaches the inner ear. This is how
labyrinthitis ossificans is caused in a patient with
meningitis.

Otology Operative surgery

1. For grommet incision where will you site the
   incision ?

   What should be the direction of the incision ?

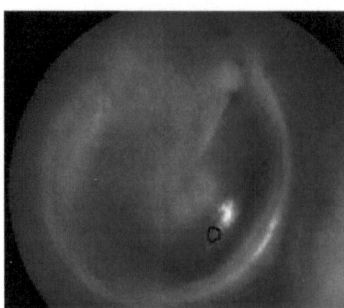

Grommet should always be sited in the
antero inferior quadrant close to the
Eustachian tube orifice for better ventilatory
function

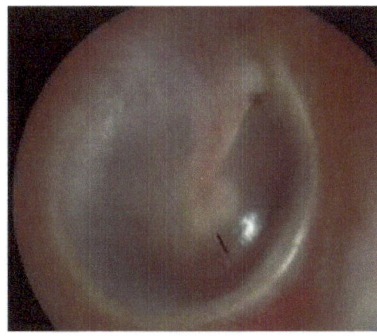

Incision should be made along the line parallel to the radial fibers of the ear drum. This will enable the radial fibers to hug the grommet in position. The drum also will heal well after extrusion of the grommet.

2.

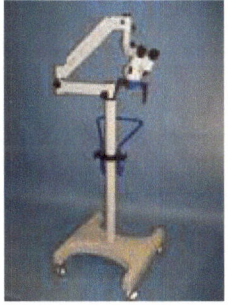

What is the focal length of the objective lens in a microscope used for otological surgeries ?

Name the major advantage of microscope in otological surgery ?

What is the of magnification used to examine the ear drum ?

200 mm

Both hands are free

6X

3.

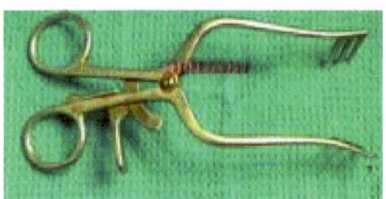

Name the instrument shown

Which surgery is it commonly used ?

Name the advantages of using this instrument ?

Mollison's self-retaining hemostatic mastoid retractor.

It is used in mastoid surgeries.

When this retractor is applied it:

Retracts the soft tissue

It stops bleeding.

Allows both hands to be free

4.

Name this instrument

Where do you use this ?

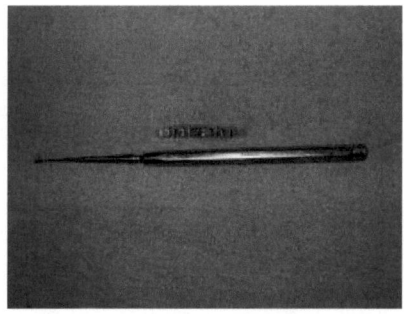

It is a myringotome. (Myringotomy knife)

It is used to perform myringotomy

5.

Enumerate the goals of cholesteatoma surgery

1. To remove all potentially erosive / invasive tissue

2. To create a smooth skin lined exteriorized cavity

3. To conserve residual hearing

4. To improve hearing if possible

6.

Name the surgical procedure

Identify the numbered structures

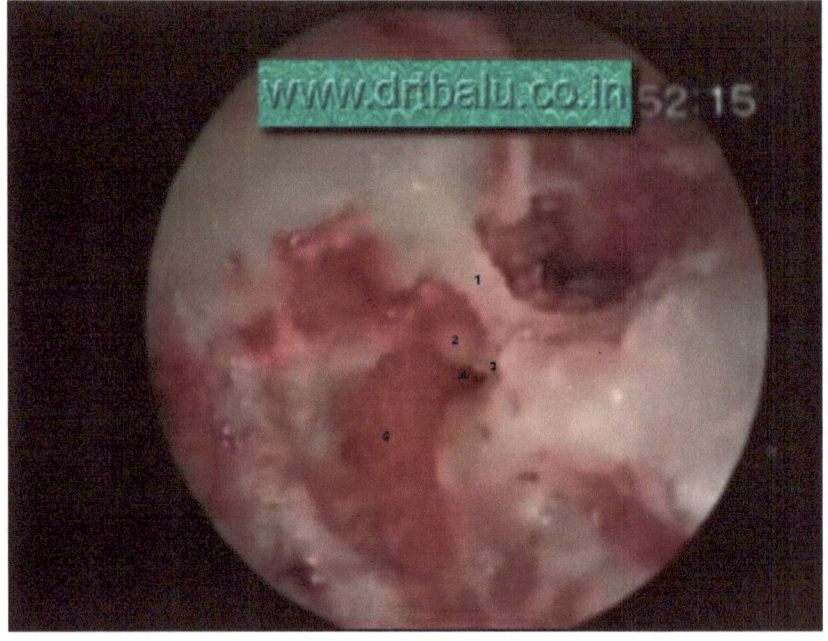

Cortical mastoidectomy

1. Posterior canal wall (bridge)

2. Incus

3. Fossa incudis

4. Aditus

5. Mastoid cavity after exenteration of air cells

7.

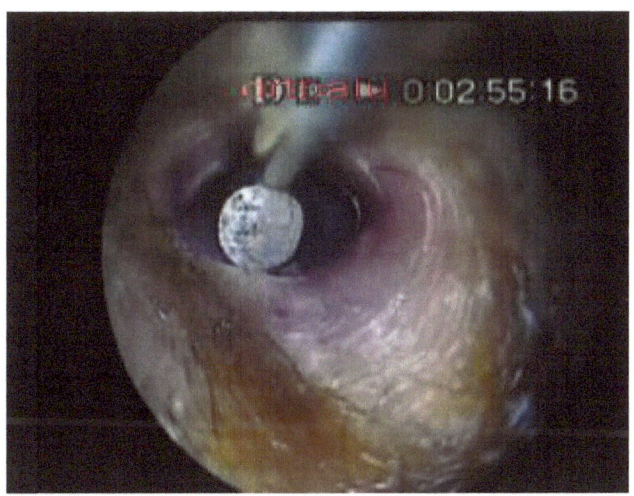

Name the incison used in this surgery

Name the instrument used

Name any two surgical procedures where this incision is used

Rosen's trancanal incision

Rosen's knife

Myringoplasty

Stapedectomy

8.

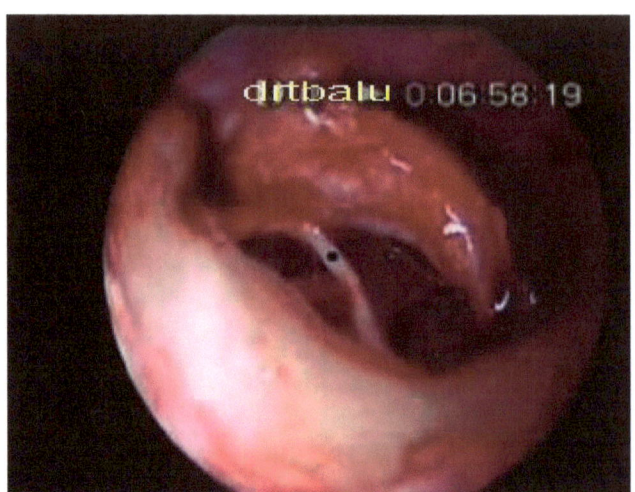

Name the flap elevated

Name the structure pointed with black dot

Which nerve's branch is it ?

Tympanomeatal flap

Chorda tympani nerve

Facial nerve

9.

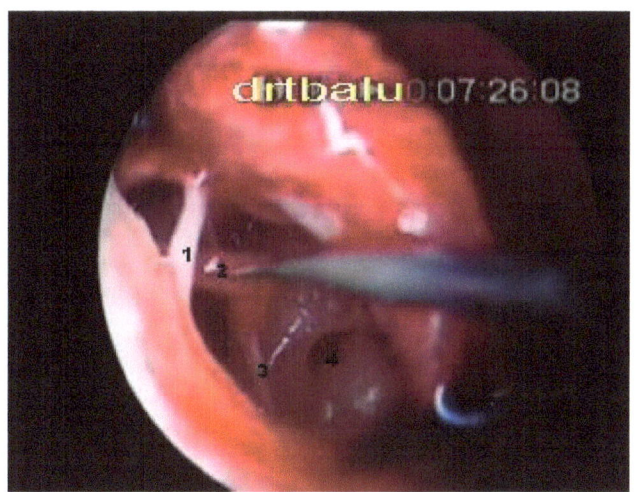

Identify the named structures

1. Chorda tympani nerve

2. Long process of incus

3. Stapedial tendon

4. Round window

10.

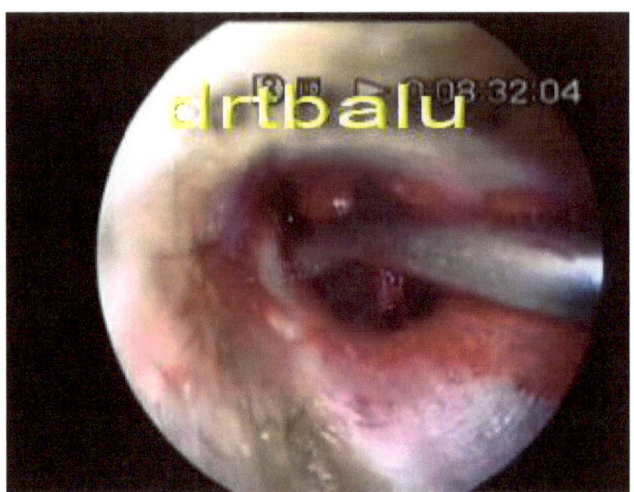

You are seeing bony over hang being curetted during stapedectomy.

How much of bony over hang should be removed ?

What instrument is used for this purpose ?

What are the dangers of bony overhang removal ?

Bony overhang should be removed till the whole of the pyramidal process comes into view.

House's curette is used for this purpose.

Incus dislocation should be guarded against.

11.

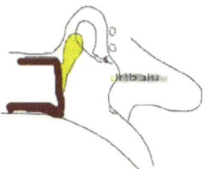

Name the type of tympanoplasty procedure illustrated

What are the prerequisites for this procedure ?

The diagram shows Type I tympanoplasty.

Prerequisites for Type I tympanoplasty are:

1. Presence of mobile ossicles
    2. Patent eustachean tube
    3. Perforated ear drum

Additional read (http://www.drtbalu.com/staped.html)

CLINICAL RHINOLOGY

1.

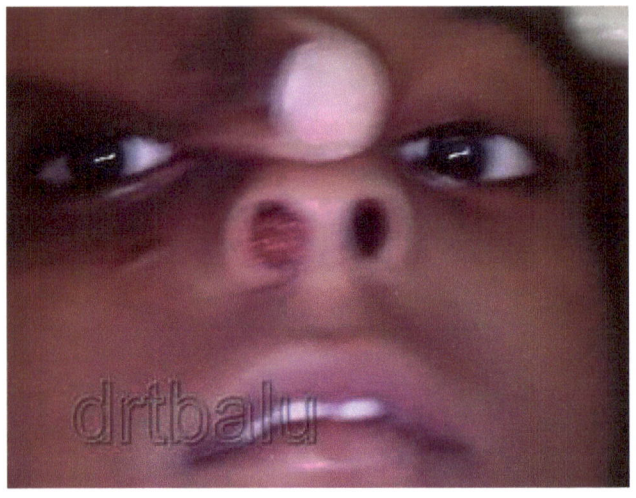

10 years old boy came with a reddish granular mass in the right nasal cavity - 4 years

He gave h/o bleeding from the mass

What could be the probable lesion ?

Name the causative organism ?

How is this disease transmitted ?

Name the drug which can be used in this condition to prevent recurrence of the same after surgery

Rhinosporidiosis

This is caused by Rhinosporidium seeberi (? Probably a fungus)

It is transmitted by taking bath in common ponds along with cattle

Dapsone is the drug which is used to prevent recurrence following surgical removal

Additional web resources:
(http://www.drtbalu.com/rhinosporidiosis.html)

2. Name the life cycle of Rhinosporidium seeberi

    a. Trophozoite (Juvenile sporangium) about 6 - 100 Microns in diameter

    b. Intermediate sporangium - about 100 - 150 microns in diameter

    c. Mature sporangium - about 400 microns in diameter

    d. Infective unit - Electron dense body (spore) It is about the size of a R.B.C

3.

    Enumerate the common sites affected by rhinosporidiosis

    a. Nose

    b. Nasopharynx

    c. Tonsil

    d. Eye (Lacrimal sac & duct)

4.

30 years old female patient came with c/o

Nasal block - 3 years

Bleeding from nose - 2 years

Loss of sensation of smell - 3 years

Fetid smelling greenish crusts - both nasal cavity

Rhinoscopy:

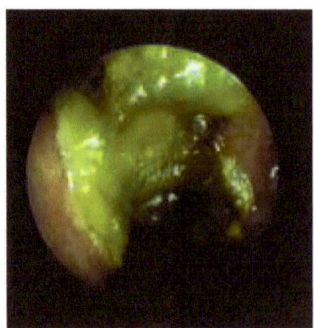

Name the probable diagnosis

Name the organisms associated with this disorder

Name a surgical procedure used in the treatment of this disorder

a. Atrophic rhinitis

b. Coccobacillus, Bacillus mucosus, Coccobacillus foetidus ozaenae, Diphtheroid bacilli and Klebsiella ozenae

c. Modified Young's operation

5. Name the constituents of Kemecitine antiozena
    solution

    Kemecetine antiozaena solution - is prepared with
    chloramphenicol 90mg, oestradiol dipropionate
    0.64mg, vitamin D2 900 IU and propylene glycol
    in 1 ml of saline

6. 15 years old boy came with c/o blocking
    sensation left nose 3 years

    Discharge from left nose - 3 years

    Diagnostic endoscopy showed:

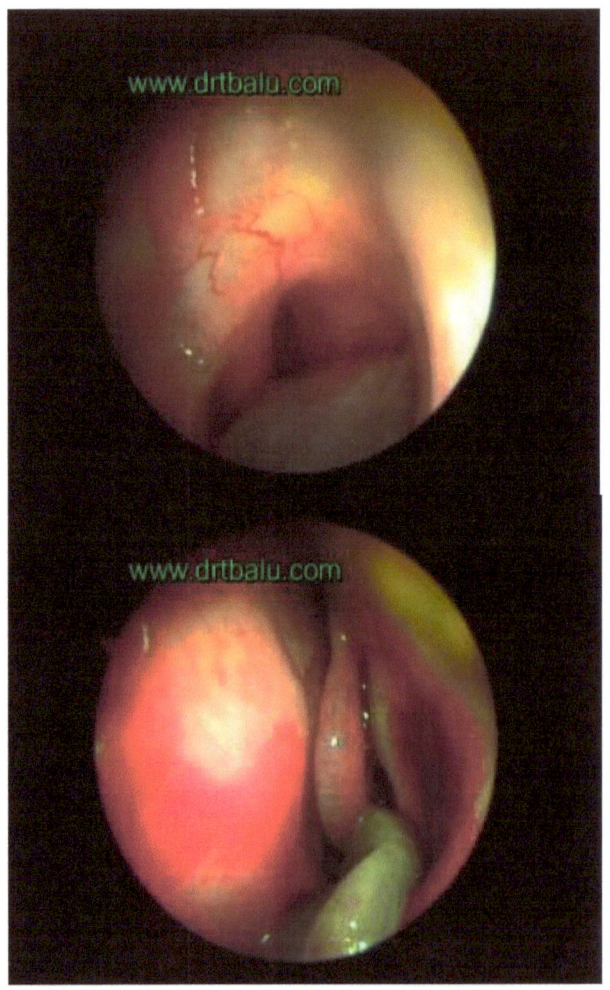

What could be the possible diagnosis ?

Why is the mass presenting at the choana ?

Probable diagnosis is antrochoanal polyp.

It presents posteriorly due to following reasons:

a. The inspiratory air current is more powerful than the expiratory current

b. The natural curvature of the floor of nasal cavity is curving posteriorly, hence gravity pulls the polyp posteriorly

c. The cilia beats towards the choana

d. The polyp exits out of maxillary antrum through the accessory ostium which is placed posteriorly

7.

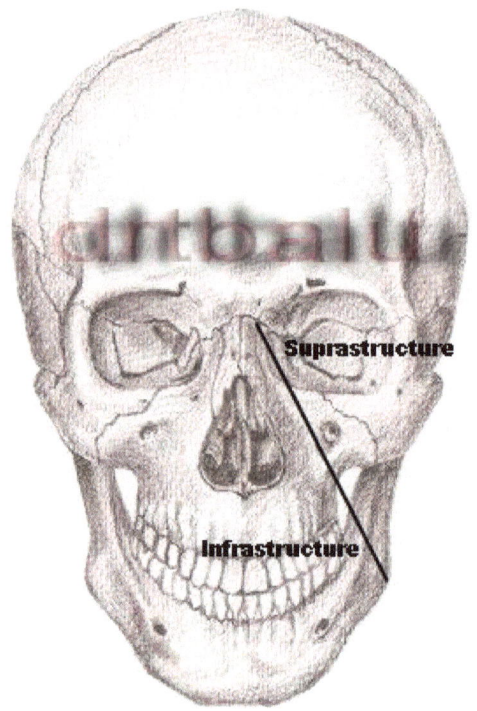

What is this line called ?

What is its use ?

It is known as the Ohngren's line. It is an imaginary line drawn from the medial canthus to the angle of the mandible.

Structures above this line are called suprastructures and below this line are called infrastructure.

Malignant lesions involving the suprastructures carry worse prognosis in comparison with those of infrastructure.

8.

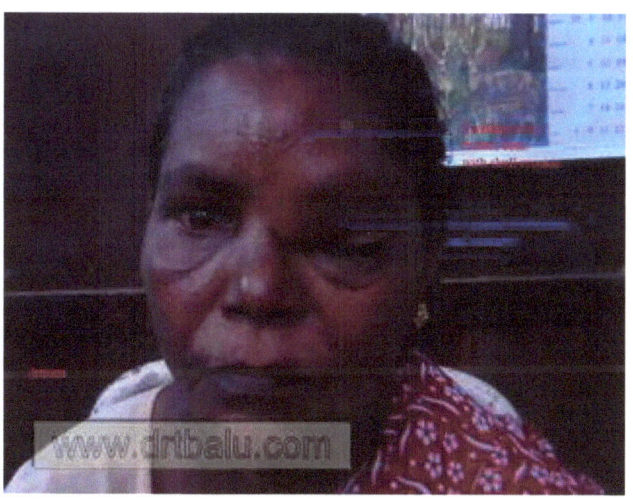

This patient came with c/o swelling over left forehead - 15 years duration

Swelling over left orbit - 20 years duration

Enumerate the clinical findings

What could be the possible diagnosis ?

a. Soft boggy swelling over left forehead.

b. Proptosis with left eye pushed downwards and outwards

c. Ocular movements full / vision normal

Possible diagnosis : Frontoethmoidal mucocele left side

9.

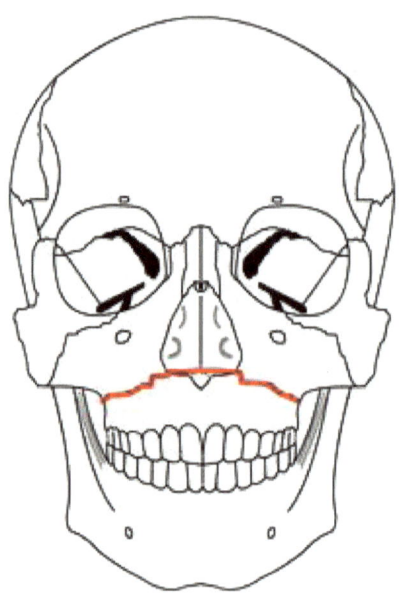

What type of fracture is this ?

Name one synonym for this type of fracture

What is the status of palate in this patient ?

It is a Lefort I type of fracture

It is also known as Guerin's fracture

Palate in these patients float into the oral cavity.

10.

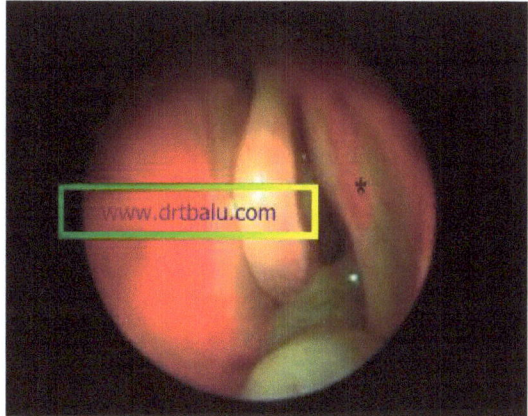

Name the structure illustrated with an asterix.

How do you differentiate this structure from the frontal process of maxilla?

It is the uncinate process. It is a boomerang shaped bone, sagittally oriented.
It is mobile as compared to the frontal process of maxilla, which is immobile.

11.

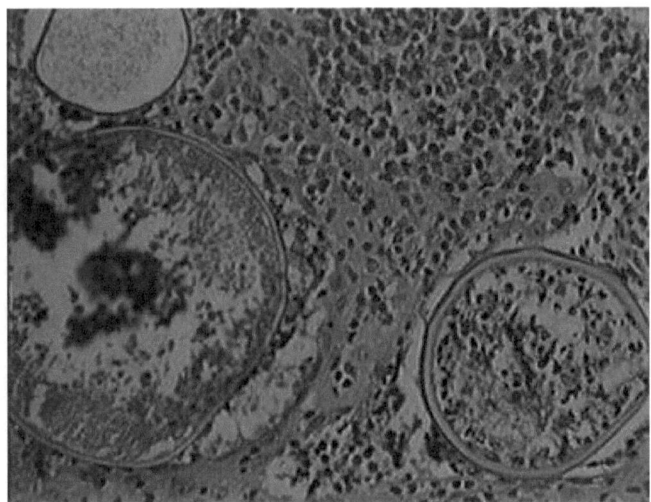

Comment on this histopathology slide.

This slide shows double walled sporangia containing spores.

Surrounding stroma shows dense collection of inflammatory cells.

Probable diagnosis - Rhinosporidiosis

12.

Name any 4 nasal complaints of sinonasal malignancy.

a. Foul smelling nasal discharge
b. Stuffiness of the nose / nasal obstruction
c. Bleeding from the nose
d. Obvious swelling over the cheek if the tumor has breached the anterior wall of maxilla / mass in the nasal cavity

13.

What is Bernhard Fraenkel triad?

What it indicates?

Bernhard Fraenkel triad include:

a. Fetor
b. Crusting of nasal mucosa
c. Atrophy of nasal mucosa

It is present in patients with atrophic rhinitis.

14.

Given below is a DNE picture of a patient.
Clinical details:
Age of the patient 18
Sex - M
C/o Bilateral nasal obstruction since childhood.
Comment on the DNE picture.
What could be the probable diagnosis?
What syndromes you would like to rule out in this patient?

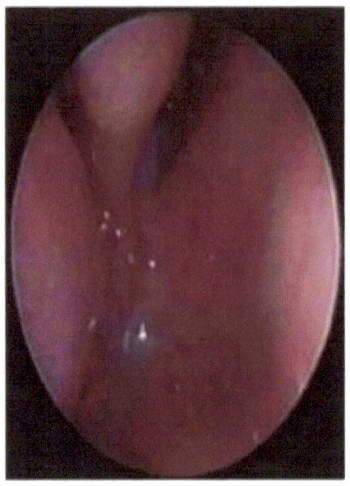

Probable diagnosis - Choanal atresia.

Syndromes to be ruled out:

CHARGE

Treacher Collins

Crouzans

Rhinoradiology

1.

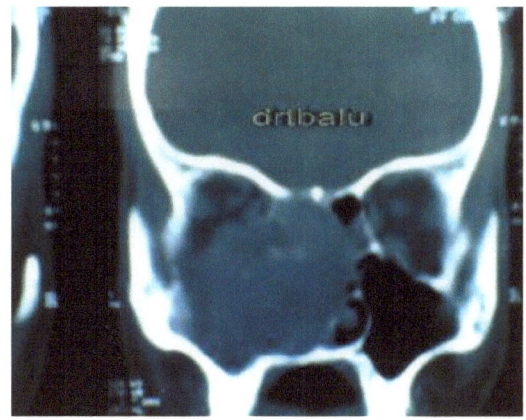

a. What view is this CT scan ?

b. Describe the lesion seen.

c. What could be the lesion ?

This is a CT scan of paranasal sinuses plain coronal view.

It shows an expanding soft tissue lesion involving the right nose, right maxillary sinus.
The medial wall of right maxillary sinus is found eroded. The nasal septum is
pushed completely to the left side. The medial and inferior orbital walls are also
involved. The mass has breached into the orbit. The skull base area appears free.

Possible diagnosis : Malignant tumor right nose and maxilla involving the orbit

2. Name any 4 risk factors for sinonasal cancers.
   a. Exposure to hard wood dust - (African Mahogany could cause adenocarcinoma)
   b. Exposure to soft wood dust - could cause squamous cell carcinoma
   c. Exposure to nickel - squamous cell carcinoma
   d. Exposure to volatile hydrocarbons - squamous cell carcinoma

3. Name 4 ocular features of sinonasal malignancy.

a. Unilateral tearing
b. Diplopia
c. Exophthalmos
d. Orbital pain

4.

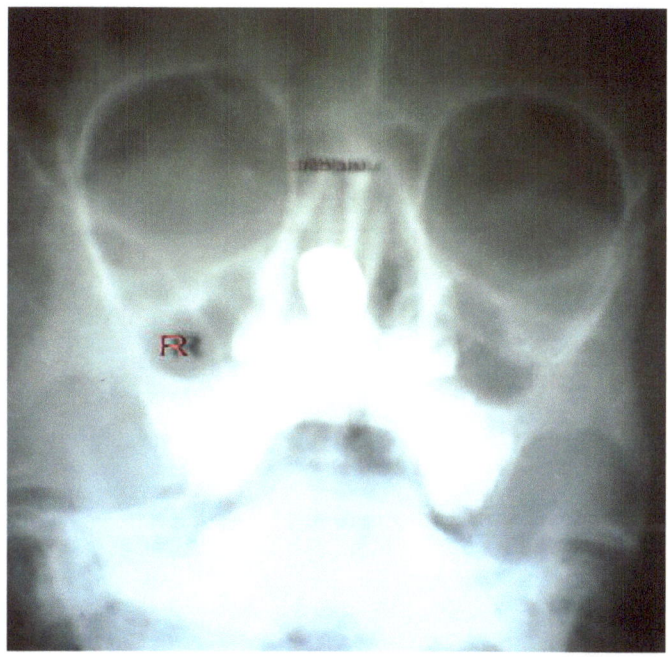

50 years old male patient came with c/o

a. Foul smelling discharge from right nose - 1 year
b. Bleeding from right nose - 1 year
c. Whitish mass seen inside the right nasal cavity -
gritty on touch.
d. X-ray of the patient is shown

comment.

This is x-ray paranasal sinuses water's view. This
shows a dense radio opaque
shadow occupying the floor of the right nasal cavity.

Possible diagnosis:

a. Rhinolith

b. Foreign body nose

5.

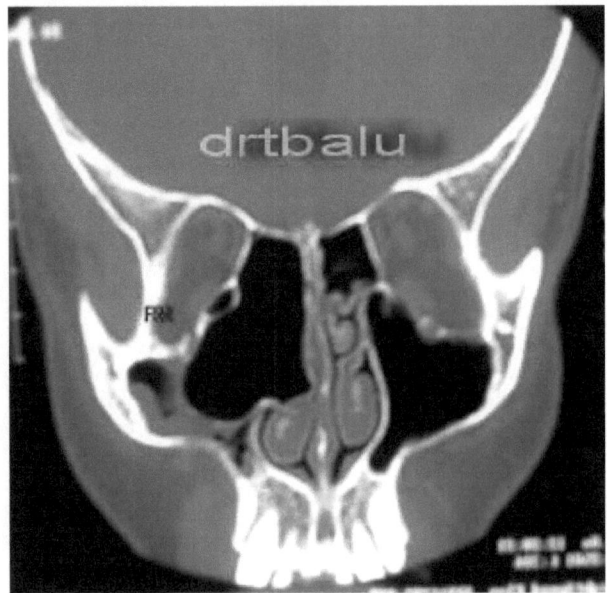

Comment on the CT scan.

This is a coronal CT scan plain of paranasal sinuses.

It shows a huge concha bullosa. The whole right
nasal cavity
is filled with concha. The concha even prolapses into
the right
maxillary sinus cavity reducing its size. The right
frontal sinus
drains into the concha. Bulla is seen in the medial
wall of the orbit.

6.

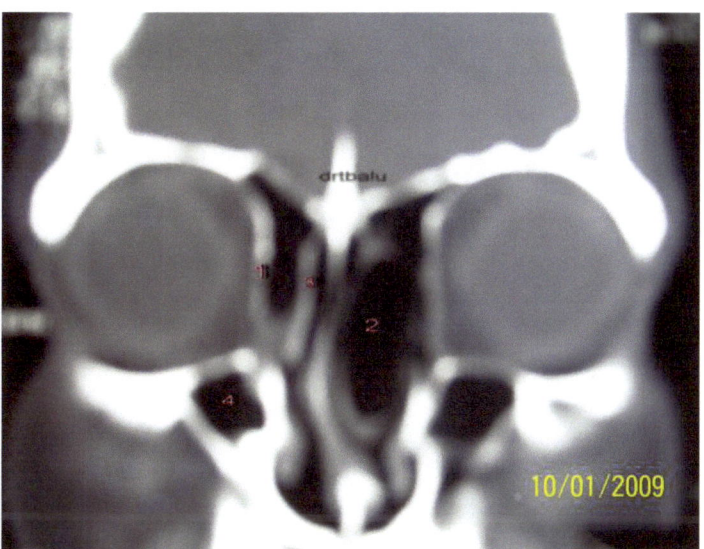

Name the numbered structures.

1 - Lamina papyracea

3 - Right middle turbinate

4 - Right maxillary sinus

2 - Concha bullosa of left middle turbinate

7.

10 years old child came with c/o nasal block both sides since birth.

Dryness of mouth since birth.

Foul smelling nasal discharge both sides.

CT scan picture showed:

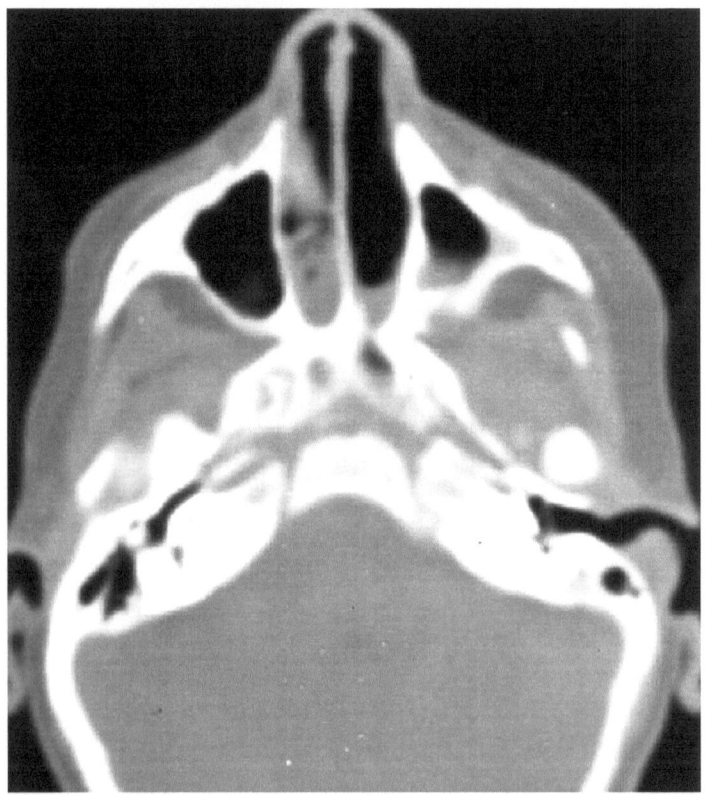

What is the view ?

What could be the probable diagnosis ?

Contrast CT of paranasal sinuses axial cut. Contrast material is instilled into both nasal cavities.

Shows that the contrast material does not flow into the nasopharynx.

The choana is closed by bony plates on both sides.

Diagnosis: Bilateral choanal atresia.

4.

Patient came with c/o double vision and swelling over right eye - 1 day duration.

H/O punched injury to right orbit ++

H/O bleeding from right nose ++

CT scan showed:

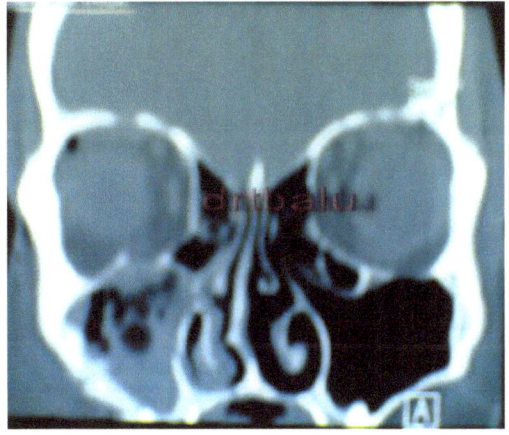

Comment on the scan.

What test you perform to rule out inferior rectus entrapment ?

CT scan shows blow out fracture of right orbit. Forced duction test is performed to rule out entrapment of inferior oblique muscle.

5.

Comment on the MRI & CT

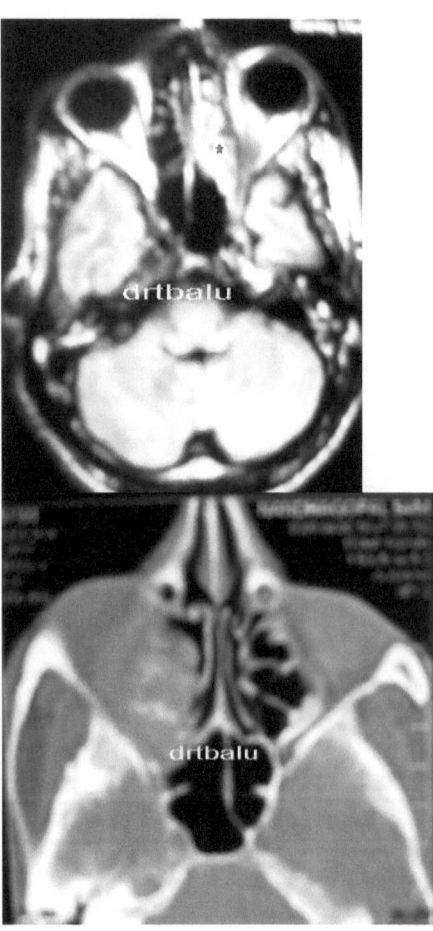

Axial MRI showing mass involving the nose, involving the optic nerve.

The mass appears bright in T2 weighted image.

Axial CT image showing heterodense lesion filling the left nasal cavity.

Left lamina papyracea appears breached.

Probable diagnosis: Fungal sinusitis with orbital complication

6.

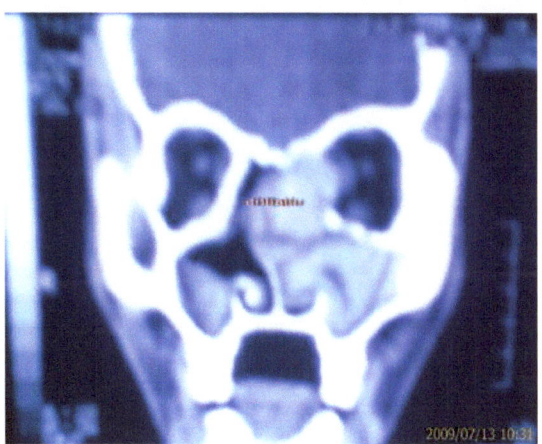

Read the CT scan

This is CT scan plain coronal view.

Heterodense mass seen occupying the left maxillary sinus eroding the medial wall of maxilla and protruding into the nasal cavity.

Anterolateral wall of maxilla appears intact

Lamina papyracea appears breached. Mass could be seen entering the orbit.

Nasal septum could be seen pushed to the right side

Possible diagnosis:

a. Fungal sinusitis.
This is considered due to the fact that the mass appears heterodense, the anterolateral wall of the
maxilla appear intact.

b. Malignant tumor of maxillary sinus (left)

11

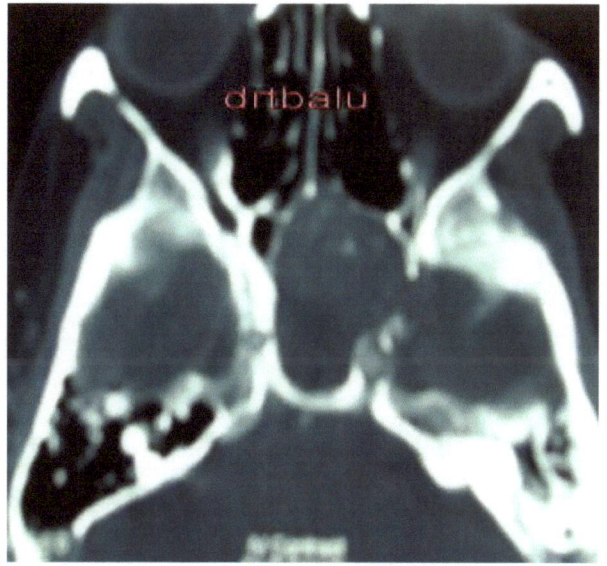

This is a CT scan of a 50 years old male patient who presented with blindness of right eye of 3 days duration. He also gave history of head ace - 1 month duration. He was a known diabetic on treatment for 10 years.

Comment on the CT scan.

This is an axial scan showing enlarged sphenoid sinus on the right side.
The right sphenoid sinus appears hazy and heterodense and **the enlarged sphenoid sinus abuts the optic nerve on the right side.**

Probable diagnosis Sphenoidal sinusitis right side.
Probably fungal in nature.

12

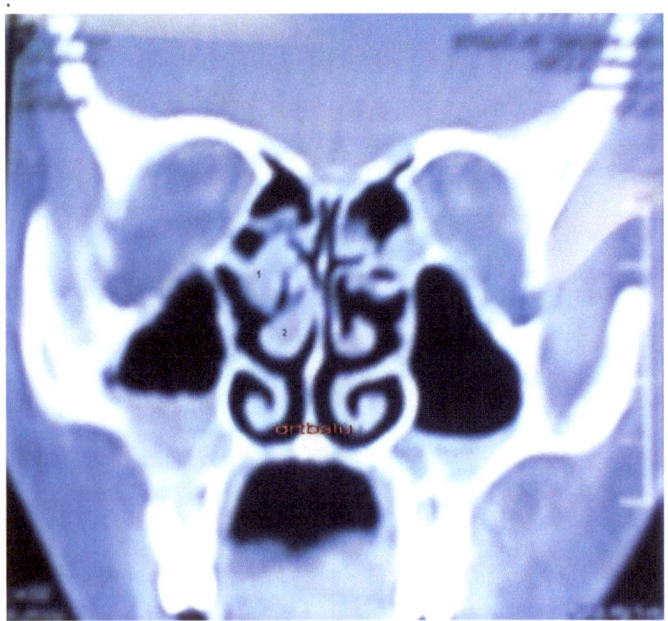

Comment on this CT especially pertaining to 1 and 2.

1 - Bulla showing mucosal thickening

2 - Concha bullosa showing mucosal thickening

Impression: Anterior ethmoiditis

13.

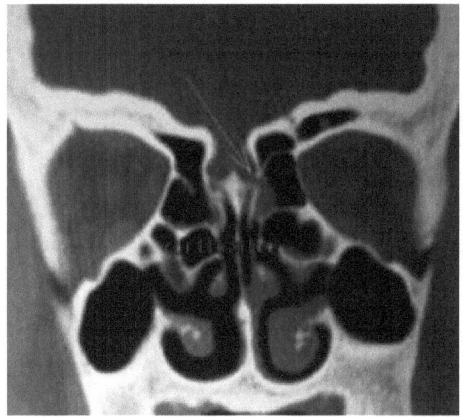

35 years old female patient came with c/o watery
discharge from left nasal cavity - 3 years
H/O fever with rigor on and off - 1 year
Head ache on and off - 1 year

You are seeing a coronal CT scan picture of the patient.

Comment on the ct.
How to manage this patient?

Coronal CT shows defect in the cribriform fossa on the
left side.
The patient is having csf rhinorrhea.
Prophylactic antibiotic therapy and closure of csf leak is
the ideal management modality.

14.

15 year old boy presented with bleeding from right nose - 1 month
Swelling just below the medial canthus of right eye - 15 days
Anterior rhinoscopy showed reddish friable mass occupying the right inferior meatus.
CT scan coronal cut showed:

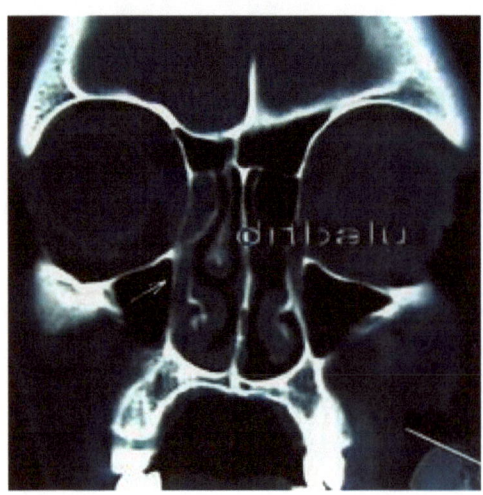

Comment on the CT scan.

This is a coronal CT scan of nose and paranasal sinuses (anterior cut).
Soft tissue shadow could be seen medial to the medial wall of right orbit.
Lamina papyracea intact. The same soft tissue shadow could be seen
extending along the nasolacrimal duct up to the inferior meatus.

Possible diagnosis: Nasolacrimal rhinosporidiosis

15.

Comment on the x-ray paranasal sinuses water's view.

What could be the probable diagnosis?

Can you comment on the status of pterygopalatine fossa from this x-ray?

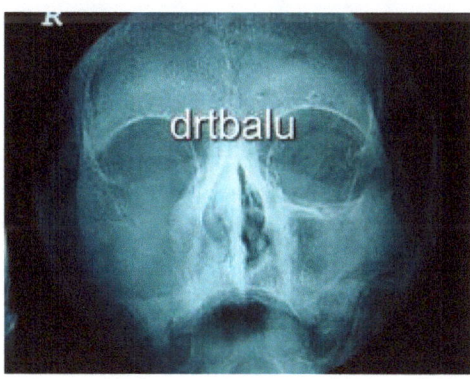

This is a digital plain x-ray paranasal sinuses water's view.

It shows an expansile lesion involving right maxilla.
Lateral wall of maxilla is found to be eroded.
The floor of the orbit (R) is also eroded with extension of mass into right orbit.
Probable diagnosis could be Malignant growth right maxilla.
Since the patient has kept his mouth open during xray,

there is no trismus and hence pterygopalatine fossa may not have been involved.

16.

Comment on the CT scan shown below:

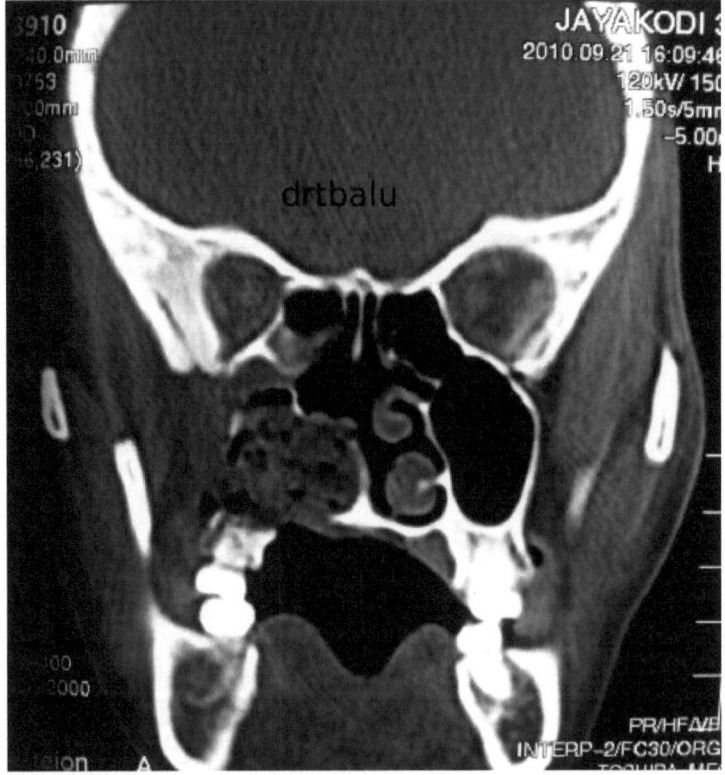

This is an image of Coronal CT plain of paranasal sinus. Posterior cut is demonstrated.
Heterodense mass could be seen arising from right maxillary sinus. Medial wall of the right maxillary sinus eroded. The same mass could be seen

filling the right nasal cavity. Hard palate
on the right side is eroded.

Probable diagnosis:

1. Fungal infection of maxillary sinus with erosion
2. Malignant lesion of maxillary sinus

17.

Comment on the CT scan shown below:

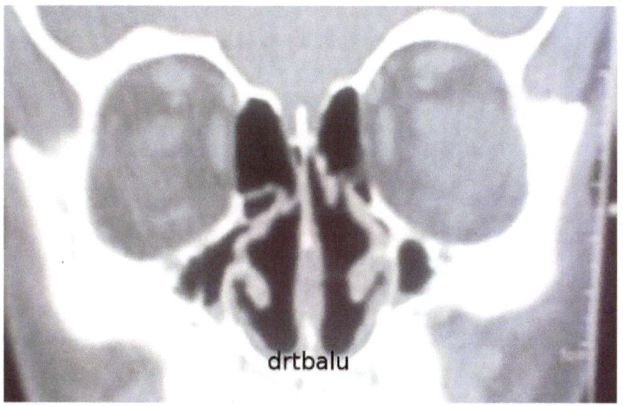

This is a coronal CT scan plain of Nose and paranasal
sinuses.
It shows thinned nasal mucosal lining.
The turbinates appear to be atrophic.
The nasal cavities appear to be excessively roomy on both
sides.
Probable diagnosis - Atrophic rhinitis.

Rhinology Operative Surgery

1.

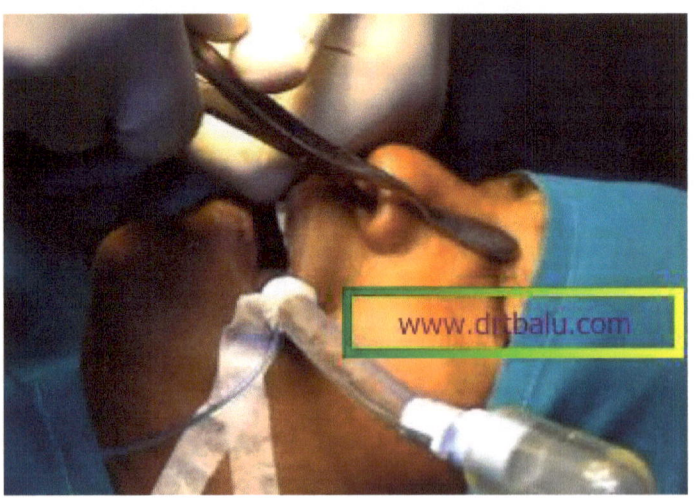

1. What is the name of this surgical procedure ?

2. Name the instrument being used

3. Name one important complication of this procedure

Reduction of fractured nasal bone.

Welsham forceps

Orbital injury

2.

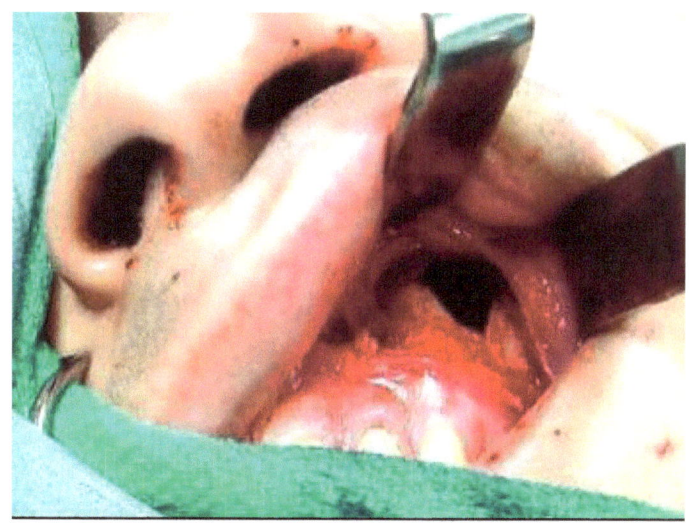

1. Name this surgical procedure

2. Name 4 indications of this surgical procedure

Caldwell -Luc's operation

1. Recurrent antrochoanal polyp

2. Foreign body in antrum

3. Dentigerous cyst

4. Oroantral fistula

5. Biopsy for tumors of maxilla

6. As an approach to sphenoid, pterygopalatine fossa, orbital decompression

3

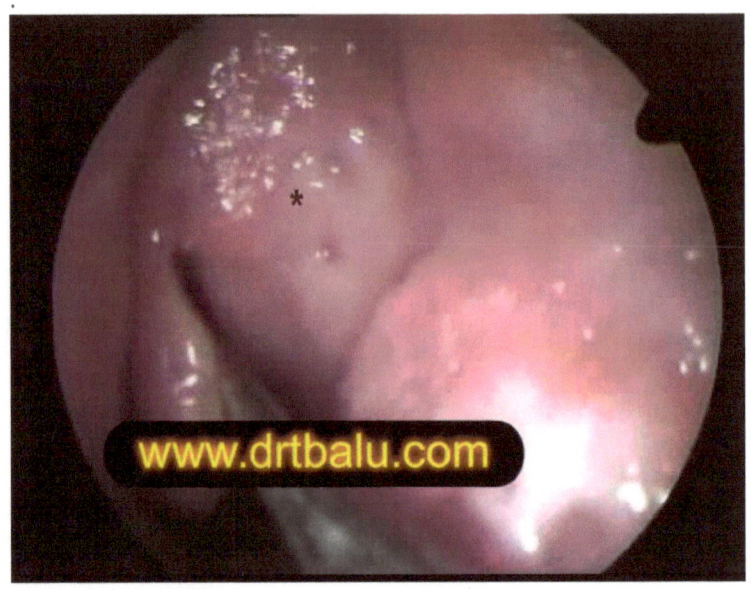

Name the structure pointed with an *

Enlargement of this structure causes __

Agger nasi

Frontal sinus obstruction

4.

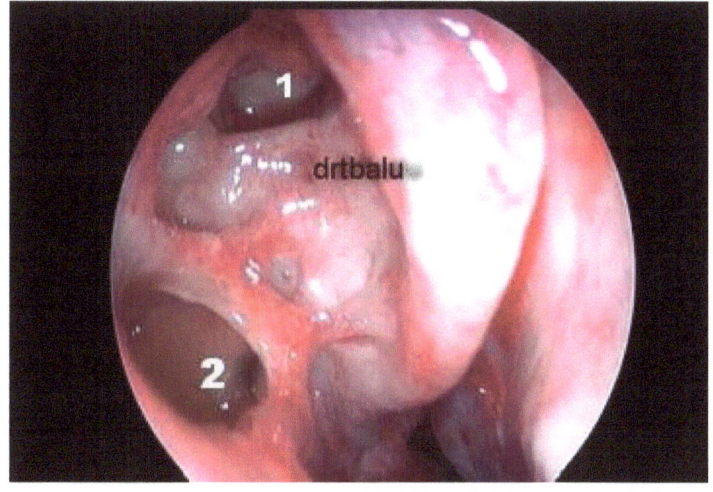

Name the structures marked 1 and 2.

1 is type I frontal cell

2 is widened maxillary sinus ostium

Clinical Laryngology

`1

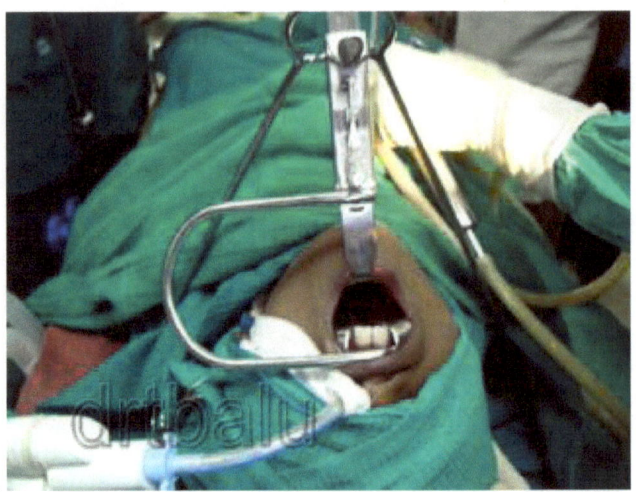

What is this surgical position called ?

Name the advantages of this position.

This is known as Rose position. This position is used in tonsillectomy.

In this position there is hyperextension of neck. This is achieved by

placing a sand bag under the shoulder of the patient. There is flexion of the atlanto occipital joint.

Major advantage of this position is that since the larynx lies at a higher

level in comparison with the oral cavity, there is virtually no risk of aspiration.

There is excellent exposure of oral cavity and its contents. Both the hands of the surgeon are free.

2.

Name the clinical importance of pyriform fossa:

1. Anatomically this is a hidden area. Any malignancy in this area would remain silent till it reaches an advanced stage.

2. This area is richly supplied with lymphatics, any malignancy in this area can easily spread to lymph nodes.

3. Foreign bodies easily get lodged here

4. Superior laryngeal nerve lies in a submucosal plane. To anesthetize this nerve a gauze piece dipped in 4% xylocaine can be placed here.

(Pyriform fossa block)

3.

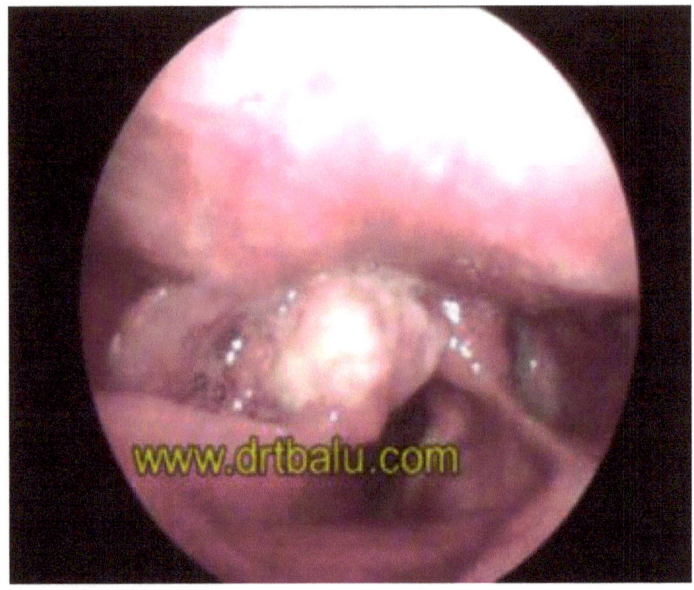

Describe this lesion

Proliferative mass seen arising from medial wall of right pyriform fossa

Pooling of saliva could be seen in the right pyriform fossa (Jackson's sign)

4.

 Name the causes of Positive Jackson's sign

1. Malignant growth involving the deep portion of the pyriform fossa

2. Foreign body being lodged in the pyriform fossa.

3. Growth involving the crico pharynx or upper oesophagus can also cause pooling of saliva.

5.

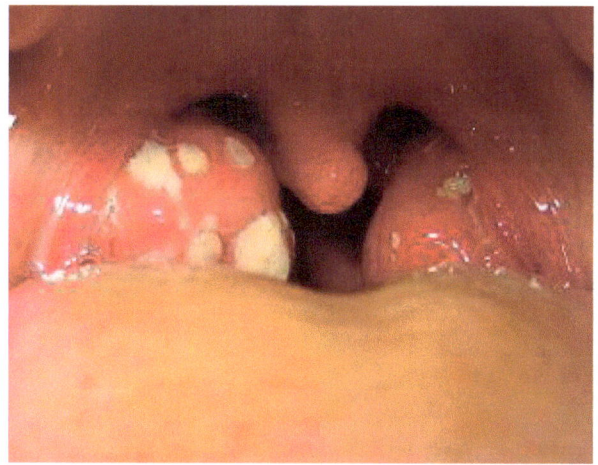

13 years old boy came with c/o pain in the throat (intense) 4 days

Fever ++

Describe this lesion.

Differential diagnosis

Acute membranous tonsillitis.

D/D:

1. Agranulocytosis

2. Infectious mononucleosis

3. Diphtheria

4. Oral thrush

5. Acute streptococcal tonsillitis

6. Vincent's angina

6.

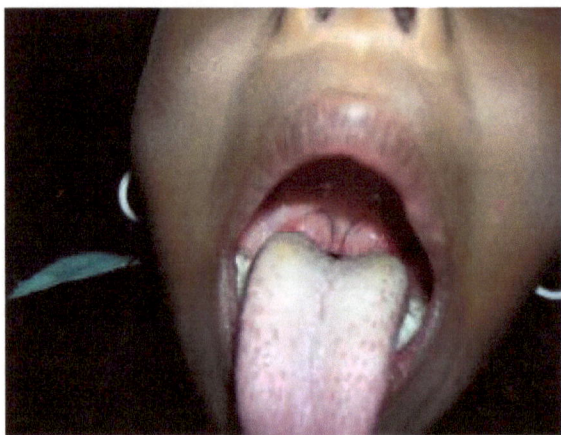

1. Comment on the grade of tonsillar enlargement.

2. Comment on the anterior pillar

Grade III tonsillar enlargement.

Anterior pillars are congested, a feature of chronic tonsillitis

7

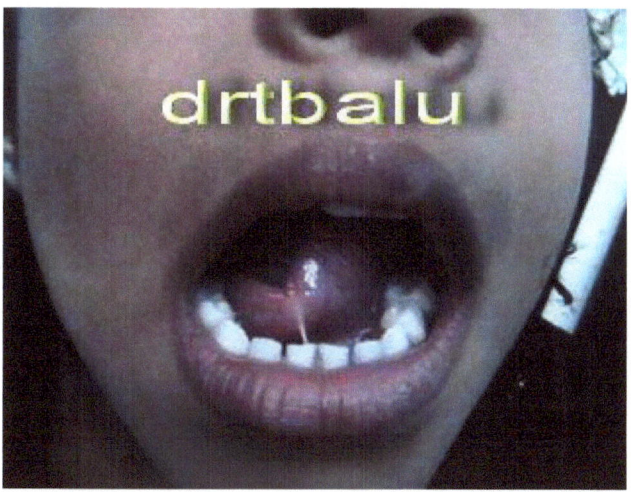

1. What is the diagnosis ?

2. How do you treat this condition ?

Tongue tie. Normally one should be able to protrude the tongue up to half way point between the lowerlip and chin.

In patients with tongue tie this is not possible as the tongue is fixed to the floor of the mouth.

Tongue tie release operation and speech therapy following surgery to improve patient's ability to speak normally.

8.

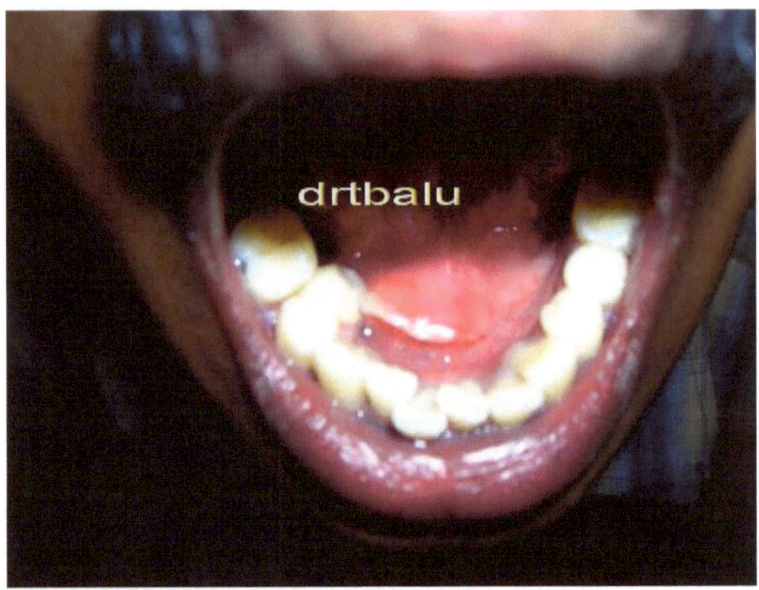

Palpate the lesion.

What could be the probable diagnosis ?

what is the treatment ?

Stony hard mass in the submandibular duct area.

Submandibular duct calculus

Excision of submandibular salivary gland.

9.

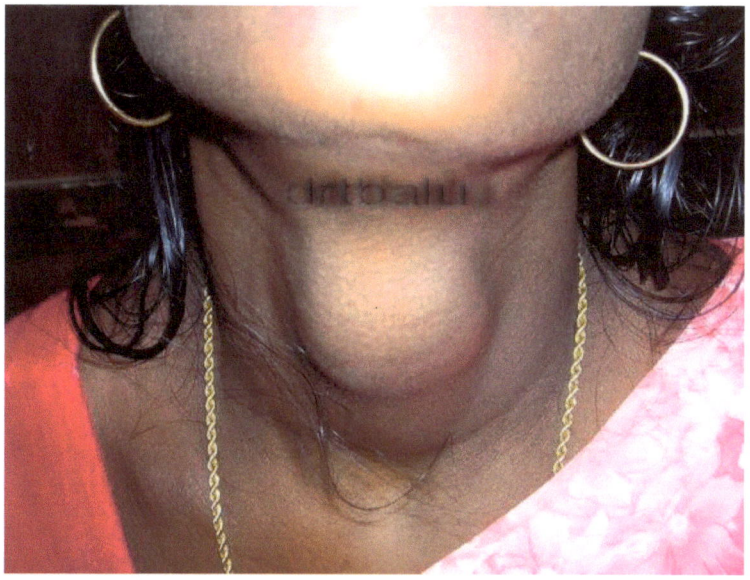

What could be the possible differential diagnosis ?

Name the clinical tests you wound do in this patient ?

Thyro glossal cyst

Thyroid swelling

Dermoid cyst

Infected lymph node

Lipoma

Sebaceous cyst

Hypertrophic pyramidal lobe of thyroid gland

On asking the patient to swallow both these swellings move upwards.

On protrusion of tongue, thyroglossal cyst moves upwards as its tract is commonly attached to the base of tongue

10.

Why is calculi common in submandibular gland?

Submandibular gland is mucinous in nature.
Its duct "Wharton's duct" is placed in a non-dependent
position (antigravity)
Parotid duct is squeezed intermittently by the buccinator
muscle, whereas wharton's duct is not squeezed by any
muscle

11.

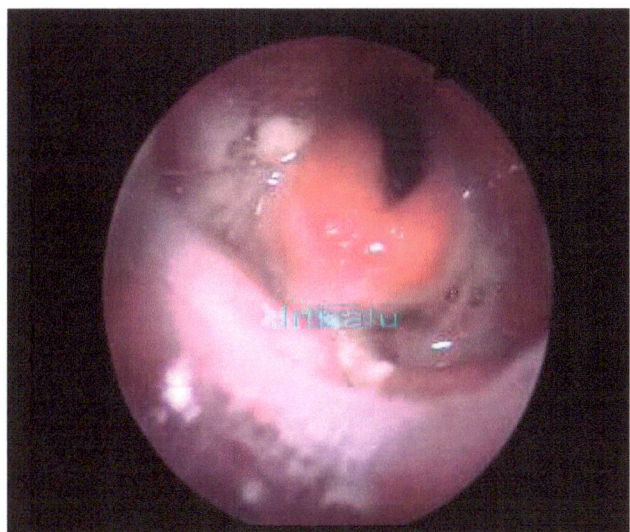

Comment on this laryngoscopic finding

What is the causative organism ?

Epiglottis is edematous and inflammed.

Haemophilus influenza

12.

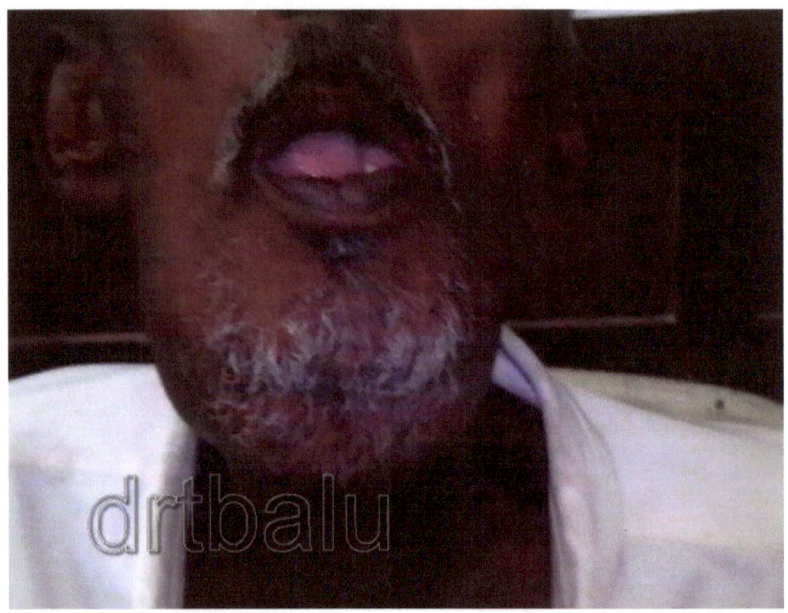

50 year old individual with c/o swelling in the floor of mouth and pain over the neck - 3 days

Drooling of saliva ++

Known diabetic under poor glycemic control - 15 years

What is the probable diagnosis ?

What are the criteria for this diagnosis ?

Ludwig's angina

To diagnose Ludwig's angina the following features should be present:

1. Rapidly spreading cellulitis with no specific tendency to form abscess.

2. Involvement of both submaxillary and sublingual spaces, usually bilaterally

3. Spread by direct extension along facial planes and not through lymphatics

4. Involvement of muscle and fascia but not submandibular gland or lymph nodes

5. Originates in the submaxillary space with progression to involve the sublingual space and floor of the mouth.

13

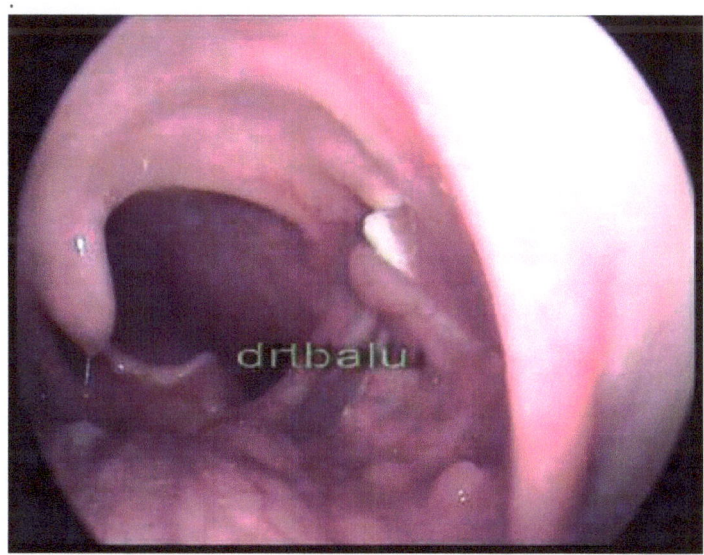

What is the white spot seen over the superior pole of tonsil ?

Will tonsillectomy help this patient ?

Keratosis tonsil.

It is known to recur even after removal of tonsil.

Mouth gargling using hypertonic urea solution helps.

14

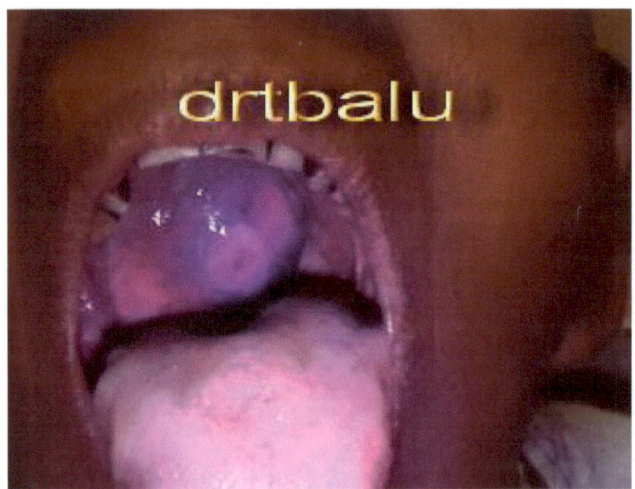

This patient came with H/O swelling hard palate - 6 years

What could be the possible diagnosis ?

Ectopic salivary gland tumor of palate

Exostosis of palate

15.

20 years old male patient came with C/O:

Change in voice - 2 weeks

H/O GERD ++

Laryngoscopy:

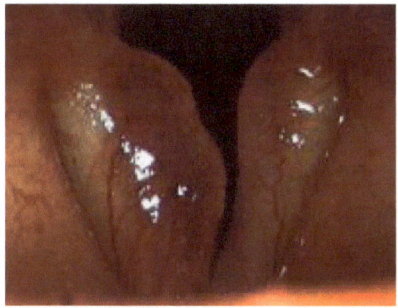

What could be the possible diagnosis?

Reinke's oedema.

Possible treatment modalities include:

Antireflux therapy

Voice rest

Surgical stripping of redundant mucosa over vocal folds

16.

This 58 years old female patient came with complaints of:

1. Foul breath - 6 months

2. Pain in the right side of throat - 2 months

3. Patient also gave history of recurrent episodes of tonsillitis

On examination:

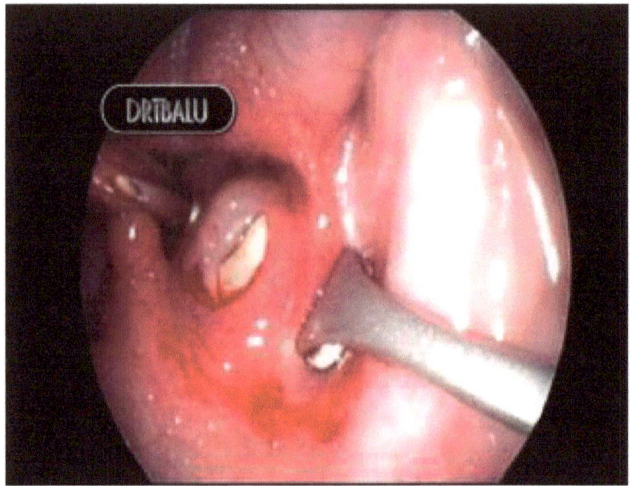

What could be the probable diagnosis?
How will you manage this condition?

It is a tonsillolith.
Unilateral tonsillectomy should be performed after treating the acute inflammation with antibiotics and antiinflammatory drugs.

17.

30 years old female patient complains of swelling in the inner side of right upper jaw - 14 years.

Progressively enlarging in size. No h/o pain or bleeding.

On examination the mass was circumscribed and hard, attached to the inner alveolar border of left maxilla.

What could be the probable diagnosis?

List out the indications for surgery in this patient

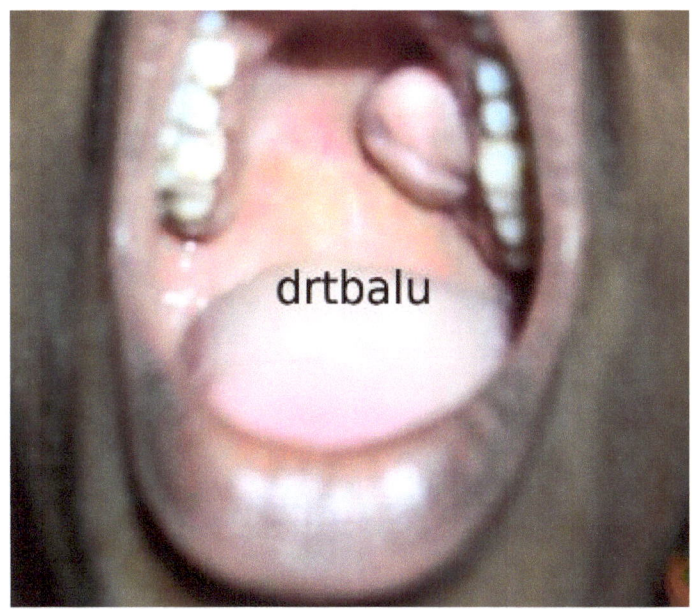

Probable diagnosis is torus mandibularis.

Indications of surgery include:

1.   Before fitting a denture
   2. Rapid enlargement of the mass
   3. As a source of autologous bone graft

18.

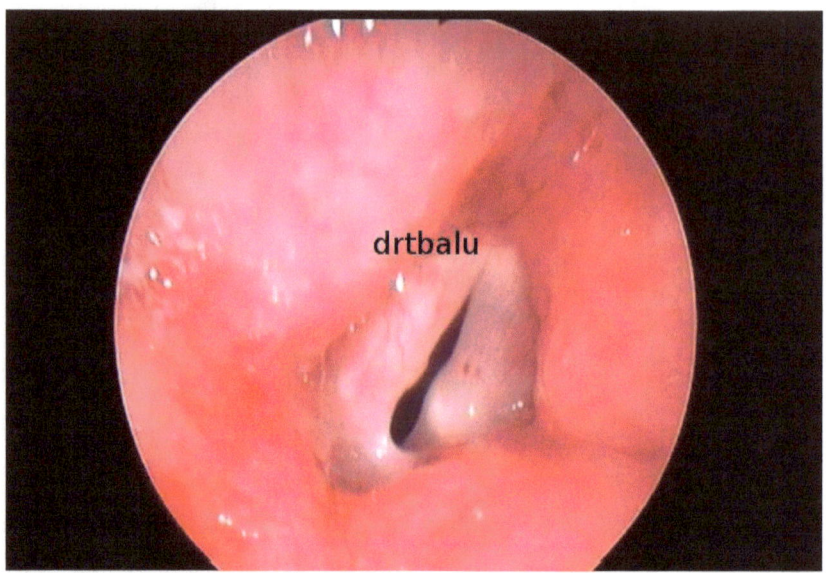

Shown above is the image captured during
videolaryngoscopic examination.

This 10 years old boy presented with tracheostomy done 4
years back for stridor.
He wanted to be extubated. He also gave h/o prolonged
intubation and ventilatory
support following a suicide attempt.
What is the ideal treatment for this patient?

The image shows posterior glottic web.

Arytenoidectomy with resection of posterior glottic web

19.

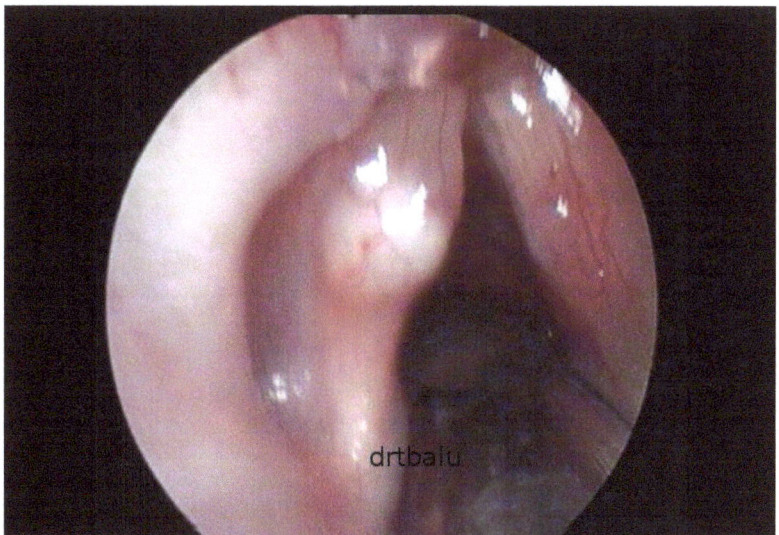

This 30 years old female patient came with c/o hoarseness of voice - 6 months duration.

She gave no h/o voice strain / abuse.

She gave no h/o repeated URI.

Videolaryngoscopic image is given above.

What is yr impression?

What could be the optimal treatment modality?

This patient appears to be having a cyst in the right vocal cord.

Probably it is a cordal cyst.

Treatment is by microlaryngeal marsupialization of the cyst.

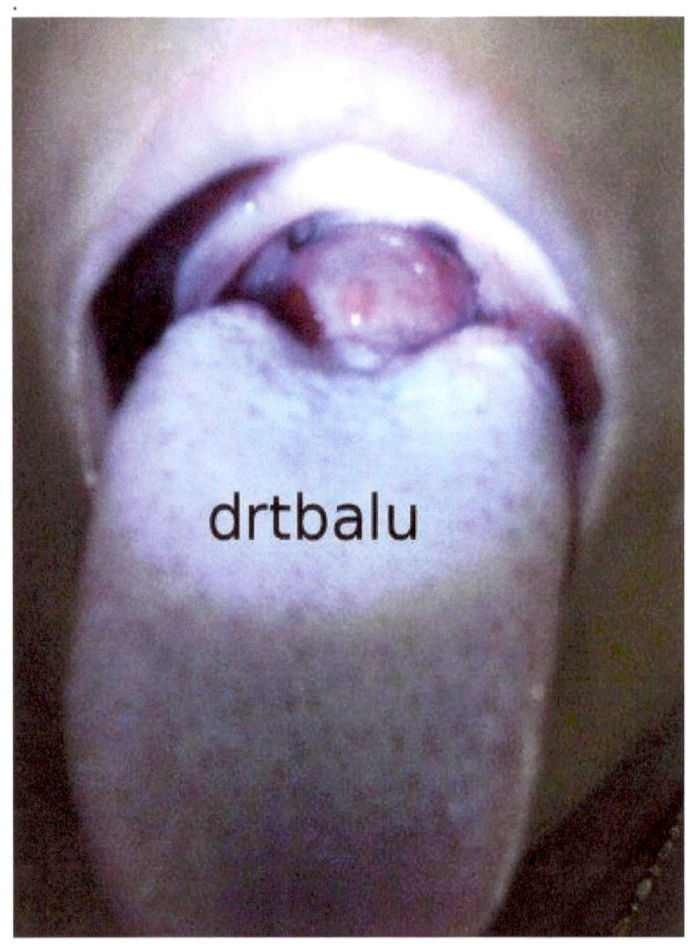

This 6 years old girl came with c/o swelling behind the tongue - 2 years duration

What could be the probable differential diagnosis?

1. Lingual thyroid
2. Vallecular cyst
3. Cystic lingual tonsil

Laryngology Operative surgery

1.

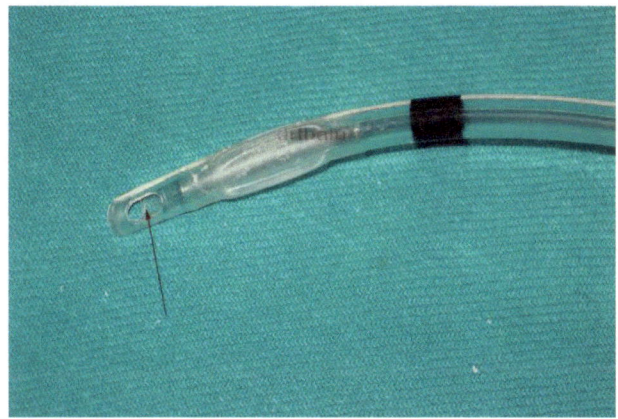

Name the structure pointed out by the arrow.

What is its use ?

It is known as the Murphy's eye.

It allows ventilation of the lung even when the bevel of the endotracheal tube is occluded.
This event commonly occurs when the bevel is in contact with the tracheal wall.

2.

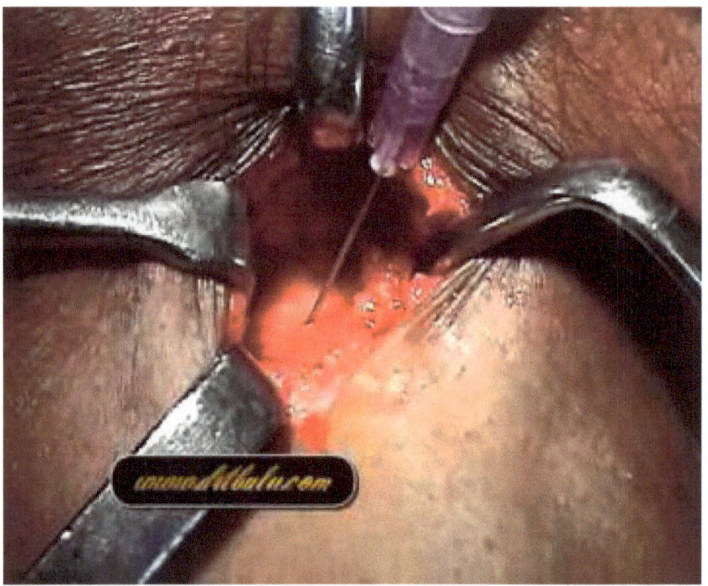

Shown here is a very important step in tracheostomy.
What is it ?
Why is it being performed ?

Identification of trachea.

This is done by injecting and withdrawing. If air
bubbles could be seen inside the syringe
on withdrawal of the piston, it confirms that the
needle is inside trachea.
The syringe contains 2 % xylocaine. A few drops of it
can be instilled into the trachea in order
to suppress the cough reflex, which commonly
occurs during tracheal incision.

3.

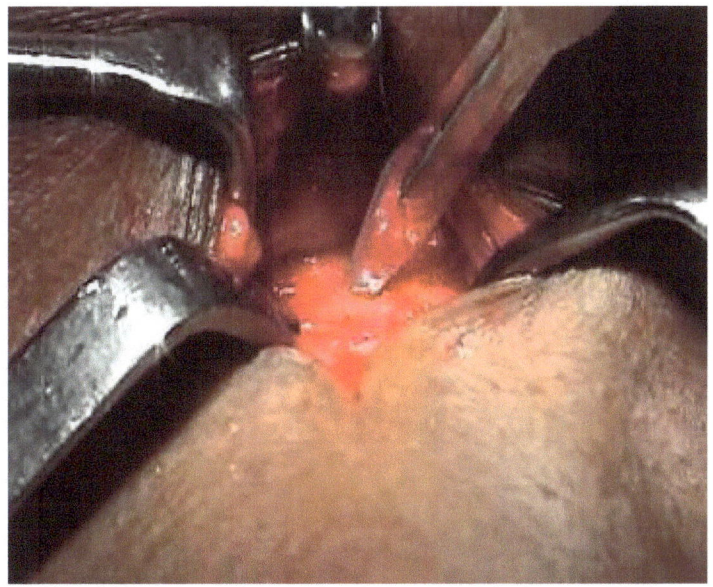

Where is the exact site of tracheal incision ?

What surgical blade is optimal for this purpose ?

Incision is sited between the 2nd and 3rd tracheal rings.

11 or 15 blade is preferred

4.

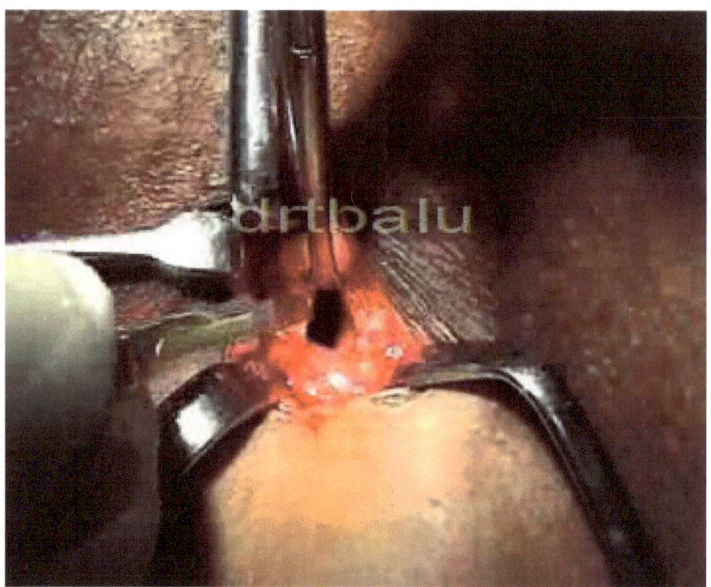

What is the name of the flap created ?

What is its advantage ?

It is known as Bjork flap. It is an inferior based flap.

Creation of this flap during tracheostomy helps to prevent tracheal stenosis

5.

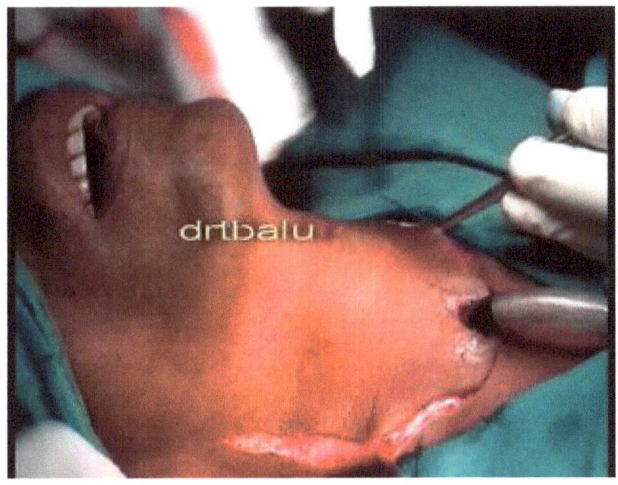

Name the incision

What is its advantage?

This is Gluck Sorenson's incision used to perform total laryngectomy.
This incision serves to separate the air passage from pharynx. The
vascularity of the flap is not compromised.

6.

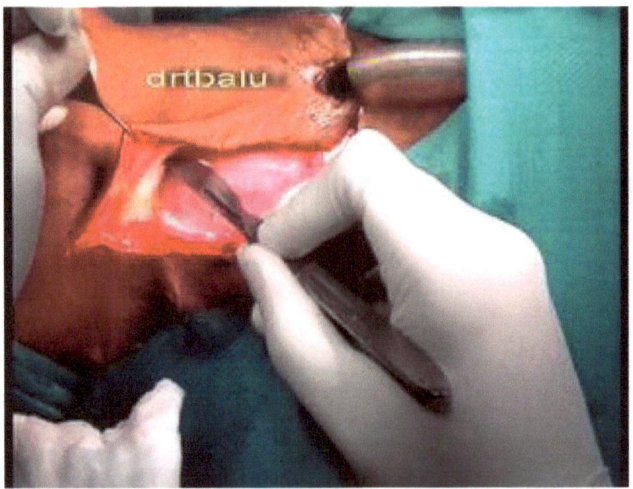

What is the plane of dissection in Gluck Sorenson's incision?

The dissection is performed in a subplatysmal plane. Staying within this plane helps
to preserve the vascularity of the graft.

7.

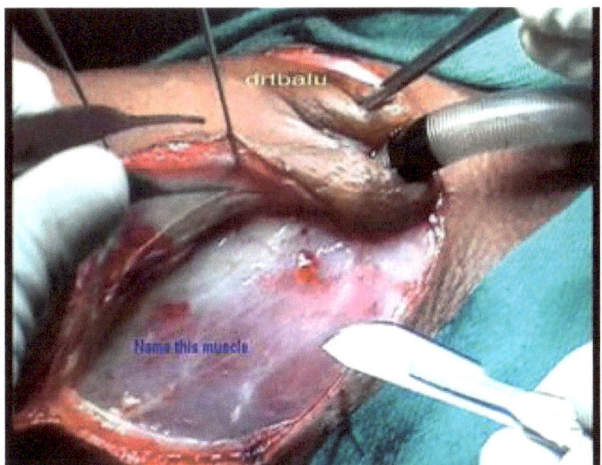

What is the muscle seen in this picture?

It is the sternomastoid muscle. Under this muscle lie the carotid sheath and jugular group of nodes.

8.

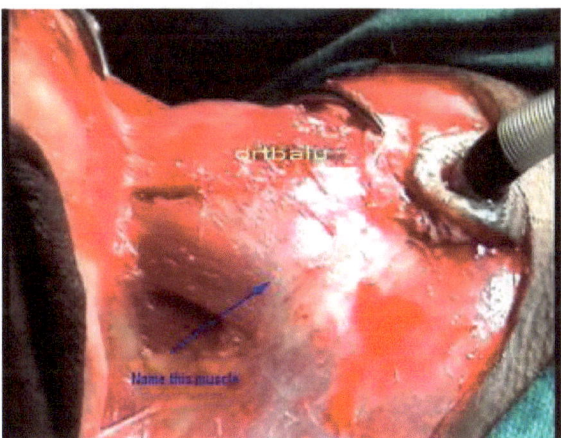

Name this muscle.

It is the omohyoid muscle. This muscle should be sectioned to expose the larynx.
This muscle should ideally be sectioned close to its sternal end.

9.

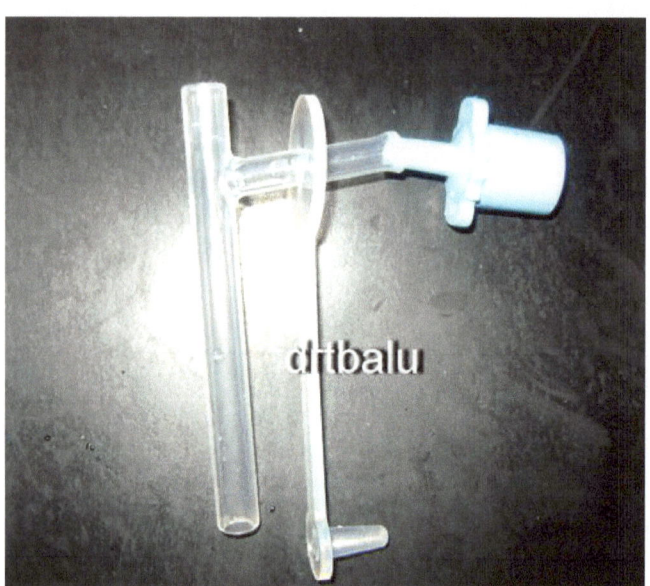

What is the name of this tube?
Where do you use it?
What are its advantages?

It is a Montgomery - T tube. This tube is made of silicone. It does not irritate soft tissues.

It is commonly used to stent the airway after tracheal reconstruction. This tube can be used for long term stenting of airway without any danger of tissue reaction / extrusion.

It has a speaking valve, and when the horizontal limb is closed the patient will be able to breath normally through the nose and speak well.

10.

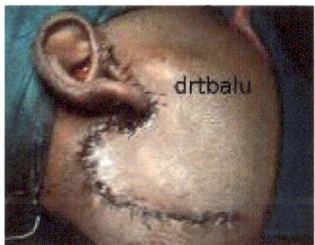

Name the incision shown in the picture.

Name the surgery in which this incision is used.

This image shows a Lazy Man S incision.

This incision is used while performing superficial / total parotidectomy

11.

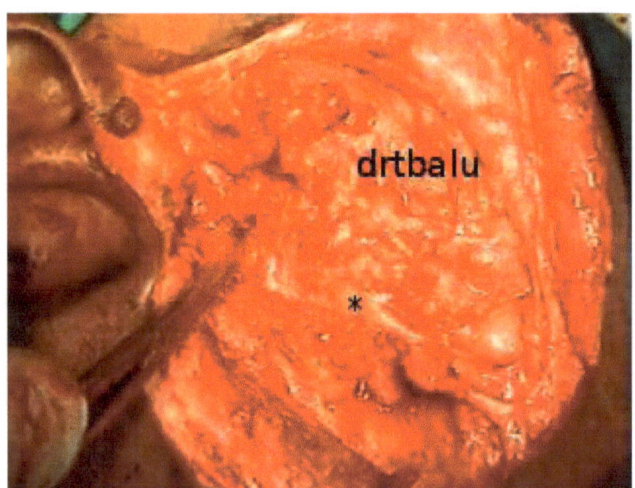

Name the structure indicated with an asterix in the above figure

It is the facial nerve seen in the parotid bed after removal of superficial lobe of parotid gland.

It is this nerve which separates the two portions of parotid gland (superficial and deep portions).

12.

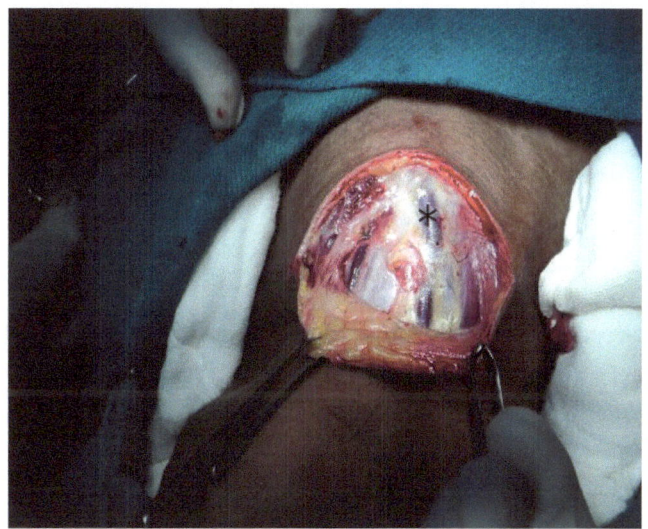

Name the structure indicated with an astrix

It is the external jugular vein. This vein can be avoided if the plane of dissection is deep to the
deep portion of the superficial layer of cervical fascia.

Laryngology imaging

1.

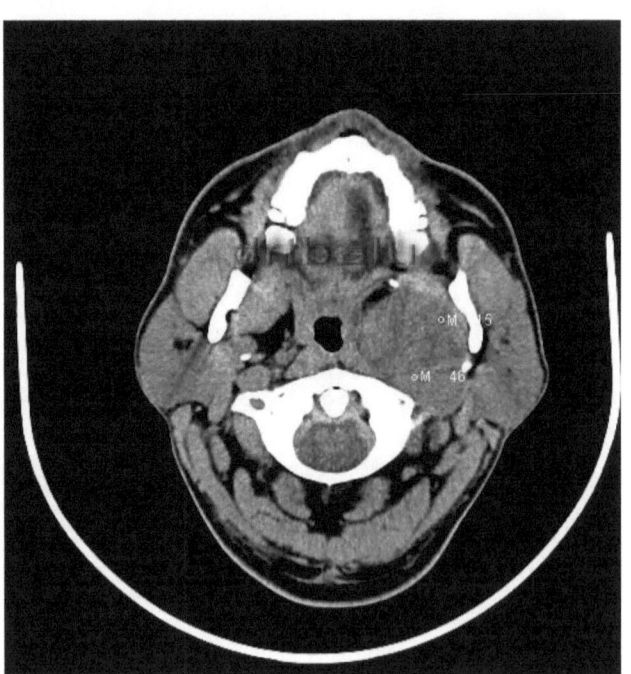

Describe this CT scan

What could be the probable diagnosis ?

This is axial CT scan of neck.

Mass seen arising from (marked m) parapharyngeal space. It could be seen extending to oropharynx.

Probable diagnosis - 1. Tumor involving the deep lobe of parotid gland, 2. Schwannomas

2.

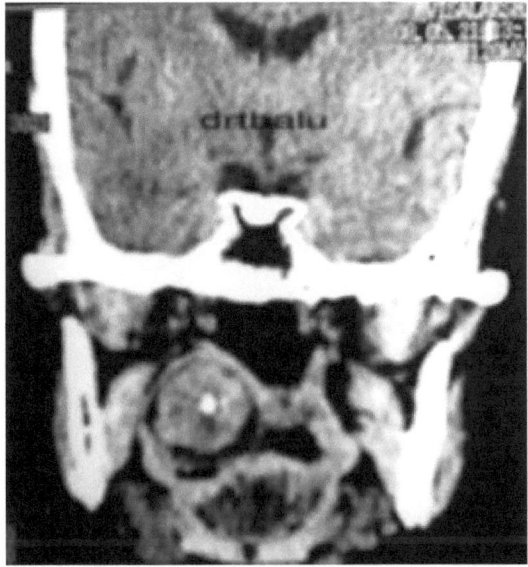

Comment on this CT scan.

This is a coronal CT plain of skull.

Spherical mass seen over the hard palate.
A small calcified spot seen in the center of the mass.
There is a clear plane visible between the mass and hard palate.
There is no evidence of erosion of hare palate.

Possible diagnosis:

? Ectopic salivary gland tumor

3.

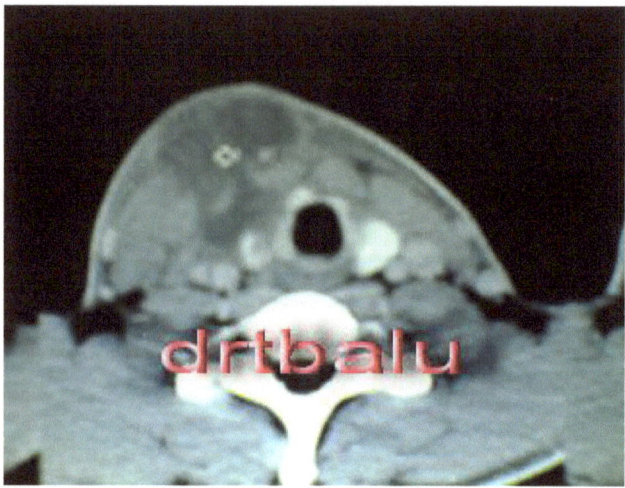

Comment on this CT scan of neck

Cystic swelling seen in front of trachea on the right side.
Probable diagnosis - Thyroglossal cyst
Dermoid cyst
Infected lymph node

4.

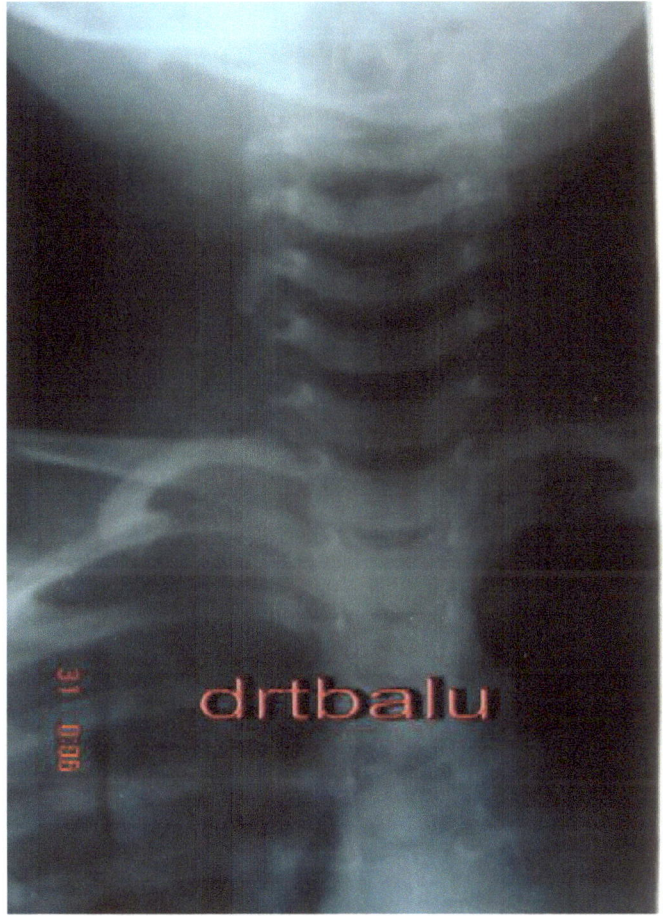

Comment on this chest radiograph

What condition could cause this?

This is known as Steeple's sign (The tracheal air column resembles the pointed steeple of a church)

This sign is a classic feature of acute laryngotracheal bronchitis.

Lateral view neck will help us to rule out acute epiglottitis, if not excluded already clinically.

This narrowing occurs in the proximal 1 cm of trachea and may extend up to the level of true cord

5.

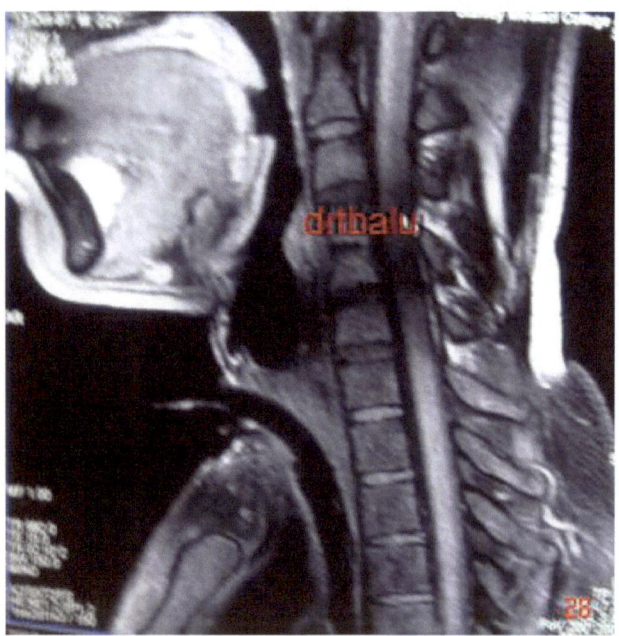

Comment on this MRI scan

What can you do for this patient?

This is a MRI scan neck lateral view.
Tracheal stenosis could be seen just below the level of cricoid cartilage.
Tracheostomy tube in situ.
Air column adequate below the tracheostome.
Resection of the stenosed segment of the trachea with

anastomosis is the treatment of choice.

Anastomosis should not be performed under tension. Tracheal lengthening procedures like laryngeal drop may be performed.

6.

Read the given CT scan.

If it is a malignant lesion what could it be?

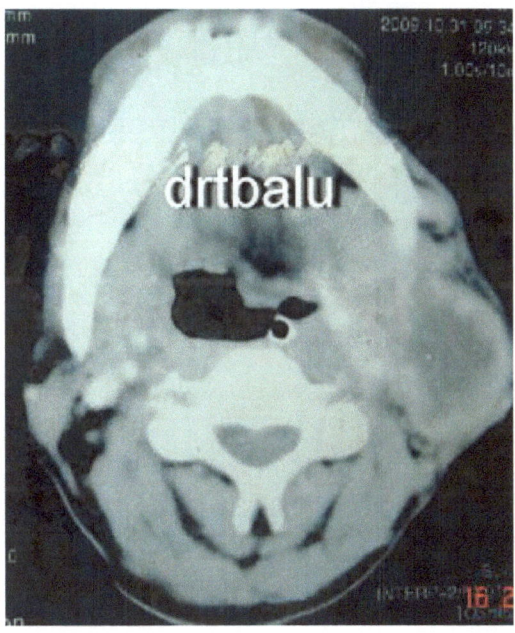

This is an axial CT scan of neck of a patient.

It shows a spherical mass occupying the lower pole of parotid gland.

The mass has a thick capsule and a radiolucent centre.

Probable diagnosis parotid abscess.

Only two malignant lesions of parotid gland are known to cause cystic changes:

1. Adenoid cystic carcinoma

2. Mucoepidermoid carcinoma

7.

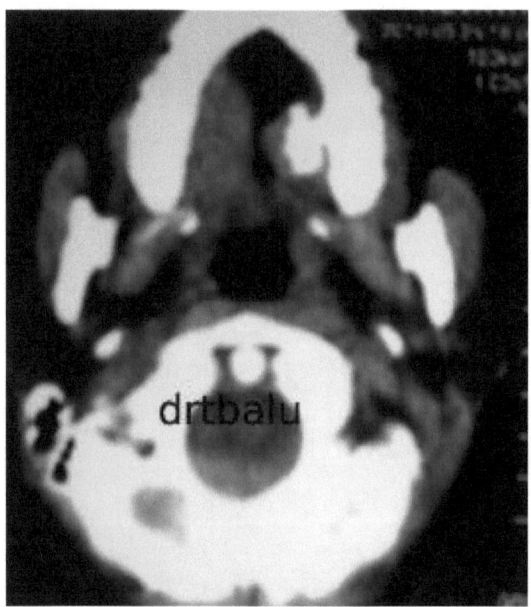

Comment on the CT scan displayed:

Axial CT of skull at the level of maxilla.
Shows a bony swelling arising from the inner surface of the alveolar border of
left maxilla. The bony swelling is attached to the inner surface of alveolar border
of the maxilla by a small pedicle. Probable diagnosis - torus mandibularis.

8.

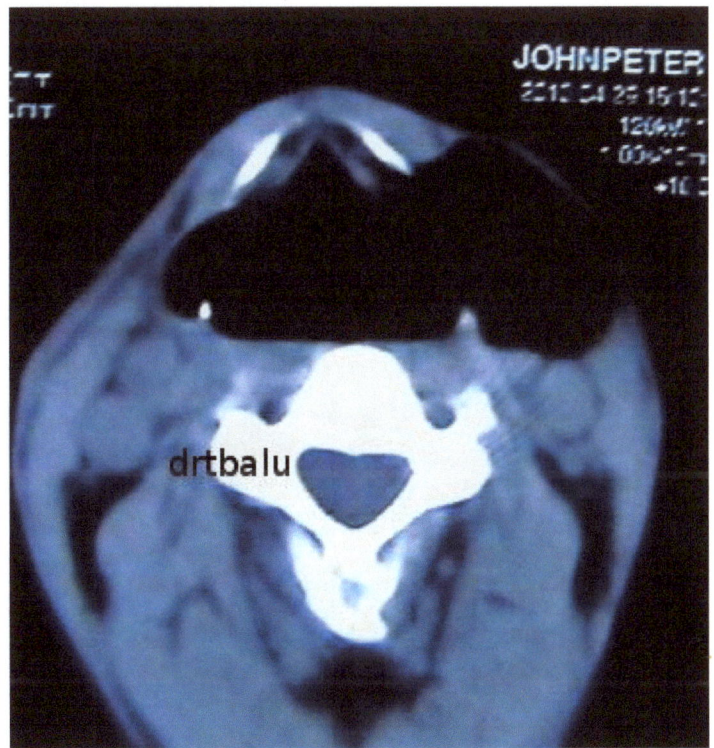

Comment on CT scan displayed:

This is a CT scan plain neck axial view showing air filled sac in continuity with laryngeal air column.

Probable diagnosis: External laryngocele

9.

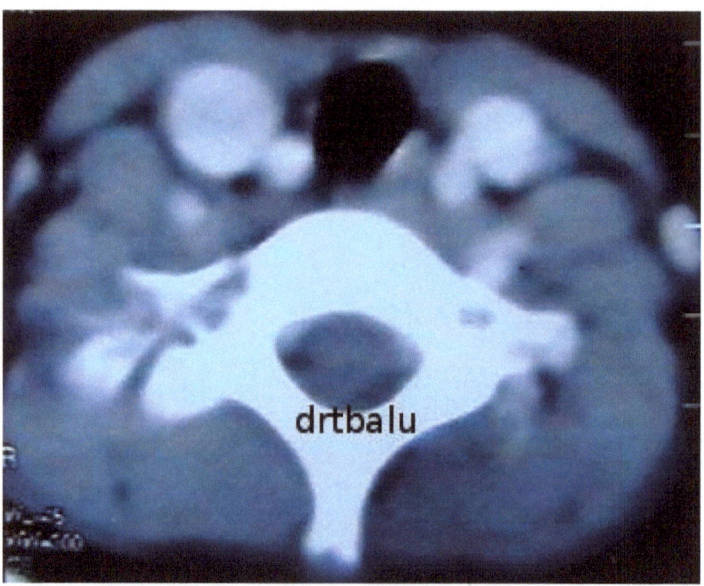

Comment on the CT scan displayed.

It is a contrast CT scan of neck axial cut.
Sternomastoid muscles seen on both sides.
Thyroid not visualised.
Carotids & internal jugular veins clearly seen
On internal jugular vein appears larger.

10.

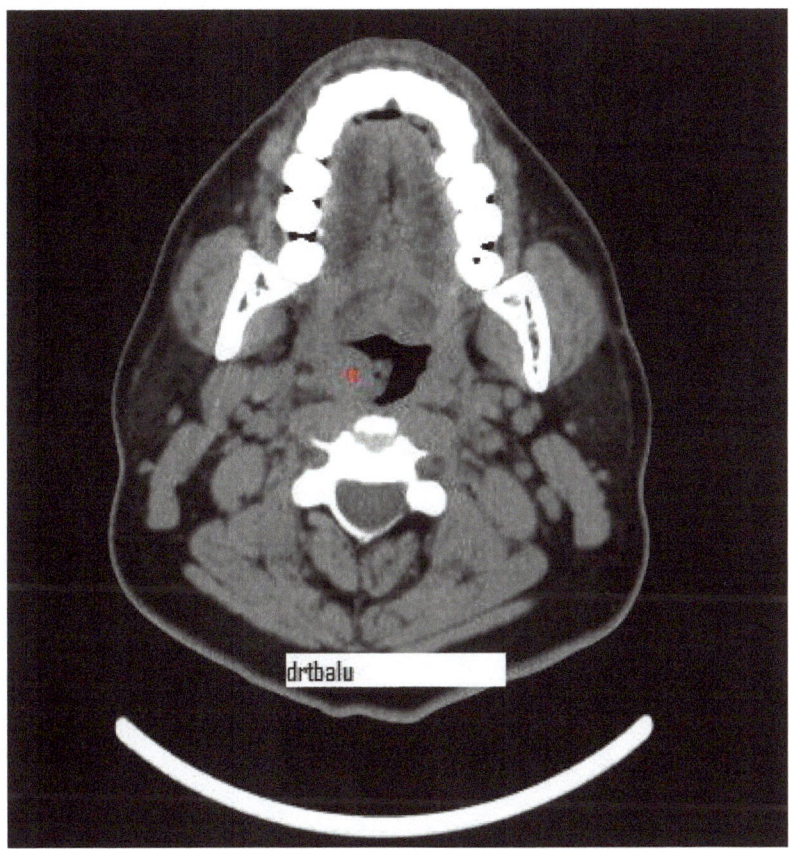

Comment on the CT scan displayed.

Enumerate two differential diagnosis for the findings seen.

This is a plain axial CT taken at the level of orpharynx.

It shows unilateral enlargement of palatine tonsil.

Differential diagnosis include:

Infectious mononucleosis

Malignancy tonsil

Benign tumor of tonsil

11.

Discuss the features seen in the x ray displayed.

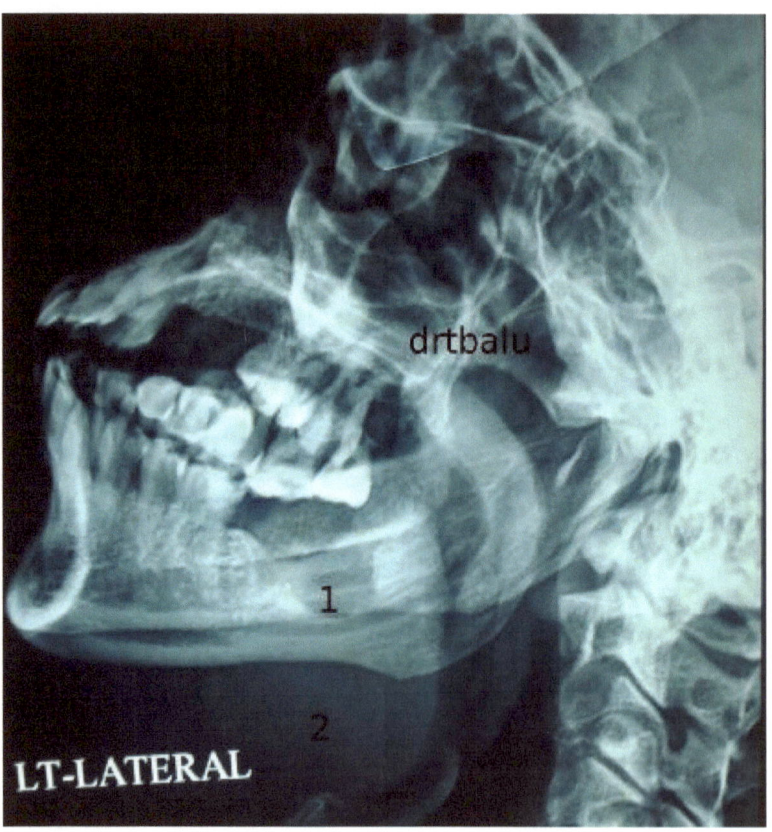

X-ray skull lateral view.

1- Radiolucent shadow under the first lower molar teeth. Probably Dental root abscess

2- Swelling over submandibular region probably Ludwig's angina

References

1. Assessment of Clinical Competence using an Objective Structured Clinical Examination (OSCE) R.M. Harden, F.A. Gleeson Medical Education volume 13, Issue 1 Pages 39-54 January 1979.
2. Critiques on the OSCE A Barman http://www.annals.edu.sg/pdf/34volno82005 09/v34n8p478.pdf
3. Patil JJ OSCE CMAJ 1993;149;1376-8
4. http://oscenotesent.wikidot.com/
5. www.drtbalu.com
6. www.drtbalu.co.in
7. www.otolaryngology.co.in
8. Radiology.otolaryngology.co.in
9. Instruments.otolaryngology.co.in